T0033016

Beyond Breast Cancer

A Mayo Clinic Guide to Healing and Wellness

TUFIA C. HADDAD, M.D. |
KATHRYN J. RUDDY, M.D., M.P.H.

 MAYO CLINIC | Mayo Clinic Press

MAYO CLINIC PRESS

Medical Editors | Tufia C. Haddad, M.D., Kathryn J. Ruddy, M.D., M.P.H.
Publisher | Daniel J. Harke
Editor in Chief | Nina E. Wiener
Managing Editor | Rachel A. Haring Bartony
Art Director | Stewart J. Koski
Production Design | Darren L. Wendt
Illustration and Photography | Mayo Clinic Media Support Services
Editorial Research Librarians | Katherine (Katie) J. Warner, M.L.S.

Contributors | Kerry R. Andrews, L.I.C.S.W., M.S.W., Alicia C. Bartz, Kimberly S. Corbin, M.D., Stacy D. D'Andre, M.D., Christina A. Dilaveri, M.D., Shawna L. Ehlers, Ph.D., L.P., Robert T. Fazzio, M.D., Ph.D., Christin A. Harless, M.D., James W. Jakub, M.D., Zaraq Khan, M.B.B.S., Janae L. Kirsch, Ph.D., Christine L. Klassen, M.D., Carol L. Kuhle, D.O., M.P.H., Heather L. LaBruna, Roberto A. Leon Ferre, M.D., Lisa K. Muenkel, Dawn M. Mussallem, D.O., Deirdre R. Pachman, M.D., Deanne (Dee) R. Smith, APRN, C.N.P., M.S.N., Jasmine D. Souers, Daniela L. Stan, M.D., Amye J. Tevaarwerk, M.D., Jesse L. VanDeWalker, Jennifer A. Vencill, Ph.D., L.P., Laura M. Waxman

Additional contributions from Creative Management Partners, LLC, and Rath Indexing

Image Credits All photographs and illustrations are copyright of Mayo Foundation for Medical Education and Research (MFMER).

Published by Mayo Clinic Press

For bulk sales to employers, member groups and health-related companies, contact Mayo Clinic, 200 First St. SW, Rochester, MN 55905, or send an email to SpecialSalesMayoBooks@mayo.edu.

To stay informed about Mayo Clinic Press, please subscribe to our free e-newsletter at MCPress.MayoClinic.org or follow us on social media.

ISBN 9798887700267 (paperback)
     9798887701738 (ebook)
Library of Congress Control Number: 2023942907

Printed in the United States of America

Table of Contents

9   Preface

**13   CHAPTER 1
        A NEW NORMAL**

14   Coping with your emotions
22   Transitioning to follow-up care
24   You've got this

**27   CHAPTER 2
        WATCHING FOR SIGNS OF
        CANCER RECURRENCE**

28   Understanding cancer recurrence
37   Supplemental screening
40   Dealing with uncertainty

42   **CHAPTER 3**
           STAYING HEALTHY

43   Follow a healthy diet
46   Strive for a healthy weight
49   Stay active
52   Prioritize good sleep
54   Don't smoke or vape
56   Avoid alcohol
57   Get regular health screenings
60   Maximize healthy benefits

61   **CHAPTER 4**
           LINGERING OR LATE SIDE EFFECTS

62   General side effects
72   Side effects of local or regional treatments
80   Side effects of systemic treatments

90   **CHAPTER 5**
           LIVING WITH METASTATIC
           BREAST CANCER

91   Treatment for metastatic breast cancer
95   Your emotions (and how to cope)
100   'My cancer is back'
105   Finding acceptance

107   **CHAPTER 6**
           MAXIMIZING QUALITY OF LIFE WITH
           PALLIATIVE CARE

107   Palliative care is not hospice care

111   **CHAPTER 7**
            CLINICAL TRIALS

112   What is a clinical trial?
112   Phases of investigation
113   Who should participate in a cancer
        clinical trial?
114   How can you find a clinical trial?
115   What questions should you ask before agreeing
        to participate?

116   **CHAPTER 8**
            INTEGRATIVE THERAPIES

117   Mindfulness
121   Acupuncture
125   Massage
127   Hypnosis
128   Medical cannabis

131   **CHAPTER 9**
            SEXUAL INTIMACY

132   How treatment may affect your sexual health
134   Restoring your sexual wellness
138   Boost your body image
140   Reconnect with your partner
142   Dating after breast cancer

146   **CHAPTER 10**
            FERTILITY AND PREGNANCY

147   Contraception
150   Pregnancy after cancer
154   Fertility options

159 **CHAPTER 11**
FAMILY AND FRIENDS

160   Easing back into family life
165   Supporting your children
168   Reconnecting with friends
173   A period of adjustment

174 **CHAPTER 12**
WORK AND MONEY

175   Returning to work
180   Finances in survivorship
188   Know your rights

192 **CHAPTER 13**
FOR PARTNERS

193   Give yourself time
194   Take care of yourself
200   Stay supportive of each other
203   Move forward together

204 **CHAPTER 14**
STOPPING ANTICANCER TREATMENT

205   Leaving a legacy
207   Hospice care

209   Additional Resources
215   Index

Preface

As Mayo Clinic medical oncologists who have devoted our clinical practice and research programs to breast cancer, we are honored to serve people at all stages of their breast cancer journeys. Most patients see us for our team-based approach to curative intent therapy for breast cancer or life-prolonging therapy for incurable disease. In both scenarios, our patients are survivors, and we strive to provide innovative, personalized treatment plans that minimize harm and align with individual preferences and values. Symptom management and quality of life are critical concerns within these plans.

This book covers common topics that we as a team talk to our patients about during and after treatment for breast cancer at Mayo Clinic. We discuss lifestyle recommendations, cancer surveillance, side effects management, living with metastatic breast cancer, clinical trials, integrative therapies, sexual health, fertility and pregnancy, relationships and finances. A chapter specific to the needs of partners and caregivers of people with breast cancer is also included. We hope that these discussions will be useful to you as a reader if you are dealing with a breast cancer diagnosis yourself, caring for a loved one, or helping a friend navigate care.

It is important to note that breast cancer is a disease that can impact anyone with breasts, of any race or ethnicity, and at any income level. In addition, disparities in breast cancer outcomes exist. We hope you will join us in our call for more research to address the unique needs of underrepresented racial, ethnic, and sex and gender minority patients, male survivors, and those who live in rural areas and are underserved by the medical system. In the end, personalized evidence-based medicine — tailored to individual needs — is the most inclusive medicine.

We are fortunate to collaborate with phenomenal colleagues across multiple Mayo Clinic departments, and we are tremendously grateful to those who have contributed to this book as chapter editors. We thank our writers for their tireless efforts to provide research-supported guidance balanced with words of encouragement to our readers. Finally, our patients are an endless source of inspiration, and it is in honor of them that we aspire to provide hope and healing to the breast cancer survivor community through the content, resources and personal perspectives within this book.

Tufia C. Haddad, M.D.
Kathryn J. Ruddy, M.D., M.P.H.

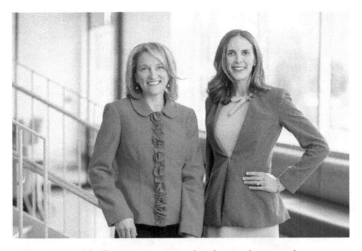

Tufia C. Haddad, M.D., is a medical oncologist who sees patients with all types and stages of breast cancer, striving to promote their understanding of their cancer and empowering them to become partners in managing their health. She has a special interest in survivorship care and works together with clinicians from many different specialties — including integrative medicine, women's health, cancer psychology, primary care and others — to provide holistic care for complex problems. Her research focuses on identifying novel strategies to transform cancer care with an emphasis on using telehealth tools and artificial intelligence.

Kathryn J. Ruddy, M.D., M.P.H., also is a medical oncologist who sees patients with all types and stages of breast cancer. She has particular expertise in treating younger women with breast cancer, helping them navigate the side effects of cancer treatment and address survivorship issues such as fertility preservation and future pregnancy. Dr. Ruddy also has expertise in male breast cancer and survivorship concerns unique to men. She is active in research focused on prediction and prevention of toxicity in patients with cancer, and finding out what patients have to say about outcomes during and after cancer treatment.

1

A new normal

As you leave your doctor's office and say goodbye to the staff, it may have started to sink in — all or most of your treatment for breast cancer is over. At last, the flurry of intense cancer treatment-related activity is in the rearview mirror. You've made it to the other side.

Now what?

"Celebrate," many people say, as if everything is now back to normal. Except . . . you may not really feel that way. Some of the side effects of your treatment may still linger. Your daily routine has changed in significant ways. Relationships may have shifted and evolved. And you've gone through emotional and spiritual changes that have left indelible marks.

The first few months after cancer treatment can be challenging. Making the transition from receiving

> My challenges returning to normal mainly showed up in finding housing to settle into. I did not understand my resistance to settling down, and always had a vague feeling it was related to the cancer that I had somehow failed to process properly. I lived in seasonal rentals for a few years, among other peoples' furniture, and finally settled into an apartment of my own. — P.M.

intensive illness-oriented treatments to no treatment or long-term management isn't always easy or smooth. You might be surprised by some of the uneasy feelings that can follow. You might even feel like the support of your cancer care team is gone. You may notice that feelings of relief are mixed with feelings of uncertainty and nervousness about the path ahead.

Adjusting to a life that now includes a history of cancer is a journey in and of itself. It involves managing a host of emotions. But it also offers an opportunity for renewal, for you to take the reins of your life and move forward in a positive direction once again.

For some people, breast cancer is still present and treatment is ongoing, both to manage cancer growth and to relieve symptoms. Chapter 5 has specific information about living with advanced breast cancer, but many other chapters in the book will be helpful as well.

COPING WITH YOUR EMOTIONS

One minute you're grateful to be alive; the next you may be overcome with worry. You're thrilled to spend less

WHAT DOES IT MEAN TO BE A SURVIVOR?

The National Cancer Institute estimates that there are over 18 million cancer survivors living in the United States today. But what does being a survivor mean, exactly? According to the National Coalition for Cancer Survivorship and the National Cancer Institute, you're considered a cancer survivor from the time of cancer diagnosis throughout the rest of your life.

Some women with breast cancer are proud to be called cancer survivors. Others, not so much. They would rather emphasize different aspects of their identity.

For ease of reading this book, we use the term *survivor* as defined above. But there's no right or wrong way to view survivorship.

time at medical appointments, but you miss the comforting support of your cancer care team. You feel enormous relief that you've made it through treatment, but you may be angry about the physical and emotional scars cancer left behind.

These feelings are very normal. Soon after your diagnosis with cancer, you were focused on getting through each day — or each moment. You may have had little time or energy to dwell on your emotions. Now all those pent-up feelings may be coming at you hard and fast.

Recovering from cancer treatment isn't just about your body — it's also about healing your mind. The good news is that feelings like fear, anger, sadness and

> I had to remind myself that it will take time to recuperate from my cancer treatments and I had to allow myself the time and space to heal physically as well as emotionally and spiritually. I continually found myself in awe of what our bodies can endure and how hard my body had worked during my cancer journey. — L.K.

anxiety often dissipate over time. It helps if you make space for your emotions and know when to seek and accept support.

Fears

One of the biggest fears you may face is that the cancer will come back. Fear of recurrence is common in cancer survivors. It can zap your concentration, make you toss and turn at night, and get in the way of relationships.

You might worry that every ache or pain is a sign of your cancer recurring. Certain experiences may cause your fear to spike, such as an approaching doctor's appointment, the anniversary of your diagnosis or news of a friend's illness.

Although it's true that cancer can recur after treatment, it's also true that most people with breast cancer never experience a recurrence. The key is acknowledging your fears and learning to put them in perspective.

It might sound counterintuitive, but a powerful way to cope with your fears is to allow yourself to feel them, rather than push them away or hide from them. Some people rely on their faith or use prayer to cope with anxious thoughts about what the future holds. Others

> My biggest fear? One word, 'recurrence.' I believe that's the biggest fear that most of us have who have been diagnosed with cancer. I also need to know that I'm still 'me' and not my cancer diagnosis. — L. K.

find it helpful to share their worries and concerns with a caring family member or friend.

Taking an active role in your health care can also give you a greater sense of control and well-being. Talk to your cancer care team about steps you can take to reduce your chance of a cancer recurrence. You can also turn to Chapter 3 for research-based suggestions for staying healthy. A good follow-up care plan, often called a survivorship care plan (see page 23), can lessen your fears, too. For more on cancer surveillance, turn to Chapter 2.

For some cancer survivors, the fear doesn't seem to get better. Instead, it seeps into every aspect of their lives, robbing them of time that might be spent focusing on work or family, or simply enjoying life. If that describes you, reach out to a member of your health care team for guidance. They may recommend a licensed therapist or a support group led by a health care professional. These options can help you manage your fears and move beyond them.

Stress
Soon after your cancer diagnosis, you might have focused completely on getting through your treatments and getting healthy. All those projects around the house and the things on your to-do list were put on an extended hold. Now they may all be competing for your attention, making you feel stressed and overwhelmed.

GRIEVING PERSONAL LOSSES

In the aftermath of cancer diagnosis and treatment, some people wrestle with a nagging sense of loss. Changes in the way you look, ongoing treatment side effects and worries about cancer recurrence can upend your sense of identity and well-being. A cancer diagnosis may also impact your relationships, career and financial health. There may be moments when you long to return to who you once were and the life you once lived.

Experiencing loss often leads to feelings of grief, which can be expressed in many ways, such as sadness, despair, anxiety, frustration or anger. Or you may experience a lack of emotion, as if you were numb.

Sometimes, it can be difficult for people who have survived breast cancer to acknowledge their grief. For example, you might feel that you don't deserve to grieve, that you should just be happy to be alive. You might be giving yourself this message or you might be hearing it from others around you. "You've survived," you may hear, "focus on your

You don't need to do everything at once. Take time for yourself as you establish a new daily routine. Try relaxation techniques like meditation or guided imagery. Consider talking with other cancer survivors. Make time for exercise and activities you enjoy. Turn to page 118 to learn about mindfulness interventions and other stress-busting therapies.

blessings, not on what you've lost." As a result, your grief may go unacknowledged.

Ironically, denying or fighting against your grief can increase its power over you. It's important to know that grieving cancer-related losses is a healthy part of the healing process. Acknowledging your losses won't make you less grateful for what you have today, but it will allow you to move past feelings of sadness, anger and frustration. Scary as it may seem, letting yourself grieve your losses can diminish your sense of grief over time.

While it's important to acknowledge and accept grief, the flip side is to become stuck in a sense of loss, especially if you find that you're frequently dwelling on your losses or if grief is affecting your ability to function in daily life. It may be helpful to share your feelings in a support group where others might understand what you're going through. Or it might be beneficial to talk to a mental health profes-sional who can provide objective guidance. If possi-ble, work with a therapist who has experience supporting cancer survivors.

Depression and anxiety
Feelings of sadness, anger or worry related to cancer can interfere with your daily life. For many people these feelings will diminish as time passes. Some research suggests that five years after treatment, the rates of depression and anxiety in cancer survivors aren't much different from what's found in the general population.

> " There are many things you put on hold while going through treatment. Afterward, you are in catch-up mode, but you have no energy. I think I have adjusted to a new normal. First, I had to stop being 'Laurie with cancer' to just being Laurie again. I stopped attending support groups as often because I didn't want to constantly be thinking about cancer. I still attend some virtual groups when the topic is educational. — L. M.

For some cancer survivors, lingering feelings can develop into or unmask underlying depression, anxiety or both. If your feelings are getting in the way of living your life, talk to your primary care provider or a member of your cancer care team. You may be referred for psychotherapy, medication or both. Early diagnosis and prompt treatment are keys to successfully overcoming depression and anxiety.

Loneliness
It's not uncommon to experience loneliness after cancer treatment. You may miss the protective cocoon of doctors, nurses and others on your cancer care team who supported you through treatment and answered all your questions. You might feel as if the people in your life can't understand what you've been through. Friends and family might be unsure of how to help you, and some people may even be uncomfortable around you because you've had cancer.

Don't deal with loneliness on your own. Consider joining a support group with other cancer survivors who may be having similar emotions. Contact your local

IS A SUPPORT GROUP RIGHT FOR ME?

Support groups, whether in your community or online, provide a great place to share your feelings and hear from others who understand what you're experiencing. But not everyone wants or needs group support beyond their family and friends. Hearing other people's cancer stories makes some people more anxious.

If you're uncertain if a support group is for you, consider whether you like being part of a group and sharing life stories with others.

If you're trying to decide whether a particular group is the right fit, consider who attends — is it breast cancer survivors only, or survivors of different types of cancer; family members; people of a limited age range? Who leads the meetings — a professional or a survivor? Is the main purpose to share feelings, or do people also offer tips to solve common problems? You might consider these other questions too:

- How large is the group?
- How long are the meetings?
- How often does the group meet?
- How long has the group been together?
- What is the format of the meetings?
- Do you have to speak or can you just listen?

chapter of the American Cancer Society for more information. Or try a trusted online message board for cancer survivors, such as the American Cancer Society's Cancer Survivors Network or Mayo Clinic Connect.

TRANSITIONING TO FOLLOW-UP CARE

Now that you've completed much or all your treatment, you probably aren't seeing your medical care team as often as you once did. But you still need regular follow-up care. The goal of follow-up care is to keep track of your overall physical and emotional health, identify and treat complications from your treatment, and watch for indications that your cancer may have returned.

Which doctor should I see?

If you haven't already done this, discuss follow-up care with your oncologist. Together you can determine whom you should see for that care. Your oncologist may continue to coordinate your cancer care, or that role may transfer to your primary care team. This decision may be based on several factors, including:

- The stage of your cancer.
- The need for ongoing endocrine or other adjuvant therapy.
- Your personal preferences.
- Your geographic location.

Once a follow-up care plan is in place, ask your cancer care and primary care teams to share their notes with one another so that everyone is on the same page.

Transferring to primary care

Having care consolidated with your primary care doctor can simplify follow up and provide you with more time to do other things. But for some people who transition to primary care after their initial treatment, the change can evoke feelings of loss or even abandonment. It can be scary to leave the safety of an entire team dedicated to your cancer treatment.

WHAT'S A CANCER SURVIVORSHIP CARE PLAN?

At the end of your cancer treatment, your care team may have given you a survivorship care plan. This document is a complete record of your cancer history that includes:

- Your diagnosis and stage of cancer.
- Details about your treatment, including beginning and ending dates.
- Possible late and long-term effects of treatment.
- Wellness recommendations, including a healthy diet, regular exercise, stress management, healthy sleep, and smoking cessation information.
- Emotional effects and support services available.
- Contact information for providers.
- Recommended cancer surveillance and other testing and follow-up appointments.

If you didn't receive a cancer survivorship care plan, work with your cancer care team to fill one out. The American Society of Clinical Oncology (ASCO) offers a free survivorship form specifically for breast cancer survivors. You can access the form at ASCO's patient information website, www.Cancer.net.

Some cancer survivors find it helpful to schedule a visit with their oncologist to help smooth the way. During this appointment, take the opportunity to go over your oncologist's recommended follow-up schedule and tests. Ask about any longer-term side effects from your cancer treatment. If desired, request a referral for mental health support or ask about recommendations for trusted support groups. Clarify who to call if you have different types of questions or concerns that your primary care doctor doesn't feel comfortable addressing.

This can also be a time to ask for a survivorship plan if you don't already have one. Take this plan with you to your follow-up appointments so you can be an active participant in your care.

YOU'VE GOT THIS

As you move on from intensive cancer treatment, it will take time to develop a "new normal." Be patient with yourself. A cancer diagnosis can change your life forever. It's important to remember that each person finds their own way of coping with the emotional and physical changes cancer brings. It's OK to feel a bit scared or apprehensive as you start a new phase of your life. There will likely be challenges ahead, but hopefully there will also be great joys in store.

> I now have a renewed sense of purpose as I approach the latter chapters of my life. I've learned to live in the moment and find joy in the little things. I've also learned not to take life for granted. I see things so much more clearly now than I ever have before. — L. K.

I HAVE QUESTIONS. WHO DO I CALL?

It can be confusing to know who to contact if questions arise after cancer treatment. This table offers a general guide, but you may also want to clarify who to contact with the members of your health care team.

Questions or concerns about . . .	Contact your . . .
Lasting or new side effects of intravenous (IV) treatments and cancer medicine taken by mouth	Oncologist
Lasting or new side effects related to radiation therapy	Radiation oncologist
Issues related to your cancer-removal surgery	Surgeon
Issues related to your breast reconstruction	Plastic surgeon
All other aspects of your physical and mental health, as well as other cancer screening	Primary care doctor
New symptoms or concerns	Oncologist or primary care doctor

POST-TRAUMATIC GROWTH AND CANCER

No one wishes to go through diagnosis and treatment of cancer. Still, positive meaning can sometimes result from negative experiences. For some survivors, the time after treatment may be marked by intense personal growth, even after a period of deep anxiety, discomfort and fear.

Psychology researchers use the term *post-traumatic growth* to refer to positive psychological change that develops from a stressful, frightening experience or trauma. Cancer researchers note that this type of growth sometimes occurs in cancer survivors. Having coped with cancer, people may discover a renewed appreciation of life, a more profound connection with loved ones, a greater openness to new possibilities, deeper reserves of inner strength or a richer spiritual experience.

Of course, not everyone feels that cancer has helped them grow as a person. In addition, personal growth doesn't preclude further stress or trauma. But if your experience has brought you new insights, don't be afraid to take them and learn from them. Such lessons can be transformative. Life can be rich despite difficulty (and sometimes because of it).

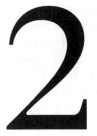

2

Watching for signs of cancer recurrence

Cancer surveillance aims to assess for cancer recurrence and catch it early when it happens. Recurrence is a major concern for many people who've finished treatment for breast cancer. Questions often come up. Is there something that you can do to prevent the cancer from coming back or to catch it early if it does? What about a new cancer? How often should you see your doctor? Which tests are most effective, and how often should you have them performed?

While guidelines are established for routine follow-up screening after breast cancer treatment, everyone is unique in their experience of breast cancer. You play a key role in your follow-up care by going to all your medical appointments and sharing any new changes to your breasts and body with your oncologist and primary care doctor. It's also important to let your health care team know your thoughts and questions about screenings and other tests. Always feel free to share with them your personal preferences and values.

Talk to your oncologist about your follow-up appointments. Figure out which health care professional to see for follow-up and who to contact if you have questions or concerns. In most cases, you will see your primary care doctor for your regular and preventive medical care. Depending on your situation, you will likely see your oncologist for a specified length of time for care that relates to your cancer treatment. If you have a survivorship plan, this information will be recorded there.

People with metastatic or advanced breast cancer may continue to receive treatment to keep the cancer under control and to relieve symptoms. See Chapter 5 for more on living with metastatic breast cancer.

UNDERSTANDING CANCER RECURRENCE

When a cancerous tumor is first diagnosed, the cancer is known as a primary cancer. Recurrent cancer is cancer that comes back after the initial treatment. Although the initial treatment is aimed at eliminating all cancer cells, a few may have evaded treatment and survived. These undetected cancer cells multiply, becoming recurrent cancer.

Recurrent breast cancer most commonly occurs within the first five years after diagnosis and treatment, but for estrogen receptor-positive cancers, it can also develop decades later. The cancer may come back in the same place as the original cancer, or it may spread to other areas of the body.

Breast cancer recurrences are divided into three categories — local, regional and distant — depending on where the cancer returns.

- **Local** A local recurrence appears in the same area as your original tumor. If you had a lumpectomy, a local recurrence occurs in remaining breast tissue. If you had a mastectomy, the cancer may recur along the mastectomy scar or the chest wall.
- **Regional** A regional recurrence is cancer that comes back in nearby lymph nodes — in the armpit, breastbone or collarbone area.
- **Distant** A distant, also known as metastatic, recurrence means the cancer has traveled to distant parts of the body, most commonly places like the bones, liver or lungs.

Recurrent cancer vs. a new cancer

If cancer is detected in the previously treated breast or chest wall, it may be a recurrence or a new cancer. It's not always easy to tell but there are clues. The tumor is more likely to be recurrent cancer if:

- The new tumor developed less than five years after the original diagnosis.
- The new tumor developed in the same area of the breast as the original tumor.
- When examined under a microscope, the new tumor cells have an appearance like that of the original tumor cells.

If breast cancer is detected in the other breast, it is more likely a second primary tumor rather than a recurrent cancer. A second primary tumor in the other breast doesn't happen very often. It's even less likely that cancer in one breast will spread to the other breast.

What to watch for
Although you'll be going through regular follow-up to monitor for any cancer recurrence, you can also watch for signs and symptoms in your body on your own. Remember that you know your body — and your breasts! — best, and you know what feels normal and what doesn't.

If you notice any of the following signs and symptoms, don't wait until your next scheduled visit. Call your primary care doctor or your oncologist. They can evaluate your signs and symptoms further, and together you can decide on the appropriate plan of action.

Signs and symptoms that might indicate
a local recurrence
If you've had a lumpectomy:
• A new lump in your breast or irregular area of firmness.
• Changes to the skin of your breast.
• Skin inflammation or area of redness.
• Nipple discharge, changes or inversion.
• Changes to the shape or contour of the breast.

If you've had a mastectomy:
• One or more painless nodules on or under the skin of your chest wall, with or without redness.
• A new area of thickening along or near the mastectomy scar.
• Changes to the skin of the chest wall.

Signs and symptoms that might indicate
a regional recurrence
A lump or swelling in the lymph nodes located:
• Under your arm.
• Near your collarbone.
• In the groove above your collarbone.
• In your neck.

Signs and symptoms that might indicate
a distant recurrence

Problems related to your bones, liver, lungs or brain, such as:

- Persistent and worsening pain, such as pain in a specific joint or back pain.
- Persistent cough.
- Difficulty breathing.
- Loss of appetite.
- Weight loss without trying.
- Severe headaches.
- Seizures.

Frequency of surveillance visits

For the first three years after completion of your initial treatment, you'll probably see your primary care doctor or oncologist every three to six months, or you might alternate visits between the two.

If you're taking a risk-reducing medicine, such as tamoxifen or an aromatase inhibitor, your oncologist

---

" Eight years after my diagnosis of invasive mixed ductal and lobular breast cancer, I honestly object to terms like 'survivor' or even 'journey,' both of which imply it's over and done. There is no way to know our actual chance of metastasis: no blood tests, no scans . . . I wonder: what does this hip pain mean? Cancer is not over. The best we can do is keep it on a back burner but remain vigilant at the same time for any signs. I don't think about it but it is there, all the time, and we adjust to it. — P. W.

will likely want to check in with you after about three months to see how you're tolerating it and coordinate any necessary changes with your primary care doctor.

After the first three years, checkups typically become less frequent. You may need to see your oncologist only every six to 12 months for the next two years, and annually after that.

If you were treated for noninvasive cancer, such as ductal carcinoma *in situ* (DCIS), your follow-up exams may be less frequent, such as twice a year for the first five years and yearly after that.

Recommended screening
Screening exams and tests aren't perfect. Generally, recurrences in women treated for early-stage breast cancer are detected because of a change in health, new symptoms or the development of a new lump. Annual mammograms can be a helpful and important tool in detecting a recurrence early, before it can be felt.

The American Society of Clinical Oncology (ASCO) recommends the following steps for routine follow-up in women who've been treated for early-stage breast cancer and who have no signs or symptoms of cancer.

Regular checkup and physical exam
Your visit will likely begin with your primary care doctor or another member of your health care team updating your medical history. They will want to know how you've been feeling since your last appointment, if you've noticed any changes in your body and if you have any concerns. They will also want to assess any changes in your general health and learn of any updates to your family history, especially regarding any family members with new cancer diagnoses.

After your doctor takes your medical history, a physical examination generally follows. During your physical exam, your doctor will check for any signs of cancer recurrence. This may include:

- A careful examination of the area where the cancer originally occurred, including the incision site, remaining breast tissue and the chest wall.
- A careful examination of your other breast or chest wall.
- An examination of lymph node areas around your armpits, collarbone and neck.

If you've had radiation therapy, it may have created changes in the structure of your breast tissue that may make breast examination more challenging (see next section).

Your doctor may also listen to your lungs for any breathing abnormalities and check for liver enlargement and any bone tenderness.

Annual mammograms
An annual mammogram is recommended for all women who have had breast cancer, except for women who have had double (bilateral) mastectomies. In addition to a medical history and physical examination, this is the only other guideline-recommended test after breast cancer treatment.

Up to 4% of women treated for early breast cancer experience a local recurrence in the treated breast. Having a history of breast cancer also increases your risk of breast cancer in general. Yearly mammograms to screen for cancer in the other breast are likely to be of even greater benefit to you now than before you had breast cancer. Evidence suggests that mammograms help find such tumors in breast cancer survivors earlier, when the tumors are still small and haven't spread to lymph nodes yet.

In the first three to five years after treatment, your oncologist may recommend a diagnostic mammogram of the treated breast rather than a screening mammogram. This is because surgery and radiation can cause changes to the internal structure of the breast. These changes typically stabilize a few years after treatment. A diagnostic mammogram adds special views of the lumpectomy area to the standard screening views and allows your care team to evaluate any abnormalities at the time of imaging. Complete imaging evaluation of these changes can help establish a new baseline for future mammograms. Once the new baseline is established, you can return to an annual screening mammogram.

Studies show there's no advantage to doing mammograms more than once a year, provided no abnormal areas show up (these might prompt more frequent examinations).

Tests that aren't recommended

Other tests sometimes used to help identify recurrent cancer — blood tumor marker studies, liver function tests and X-rays — haven't been found to be effective or useful in prolonging survival or improving quality of life. Tests that are not recommended by ASCO for detecting recurrent or new cancer in the absence of concerning symptoms include laboratory and imaging tests such as:

- A chest X-ray to check for tumors in the lung.
- An ultrasound to check for tumors in the liver.
- A bone scan to check for tumors in the bone.
- A computerized tomography (CT) scan or magnetic resonance image (MRI) to look for cancer in the soft tissues and organs of the chest, abdomen and pelvis.
- A blood test (blood tumor marker study) to check for certain substances in the blood that may be elevated in people with cancer.
- A complete blood count (CBC) to check levels of white and red blood cells and blood platelets.

IF YOU HAVE BREAST RECONSTRUCTION

Mammography isn't needed or recommended if you've had a mastectomy with any form of reconstruction. If you've had a single mastectomy with reconstruction, screening mammography done regularly on your other breast is important. Mammograms also remain important if you had breast reconstruction, including with implants, after a lumpectomy.

It is important to perform breast self-exams on your natural breast and the skin and surrounding area of your reconstructed breast. This may help you become familiar with the changes to your breast after surgery so that you can be alert to any new changes and report those to your doctor.

Some cancer clinics recommend an ultrasound or MRI in five to six years or if there are symptoms after silicone implant reconstruction. This is done to check that there's no sign of a leak from, or a rupture of, the implants. It is important to follow up with your plastic surgeon at least every few years to evaluate the breasts and changes that can happen over time.

- Liver and kidney function tests to check that these organs are functioning normally.

There's little evidence — despite multiple large studies — that these tests prolong survival or improve quality of life. In addition, these tests aren't always accurate — they may miss signs of a recurrence or, just

WHAT IS THE ROLE OF FOLLOW-UP MAMMOGRAMS IN MEN WITH BREAST CANCER?

Since breast cancer in men is rare, annual screening mammograms aren't recommended for men in general. But what about men who have had breast cancer?

In general, experts recommend that men who have had a lumpectomy for breast cancer return to their primary care doctors to prescribe mammograms of the remaining breast tissue on the affected side once a year, to monitor for signs of recurrence.

There is no standard recommendation for whether all men with a history of breast cancer should undergo screening mammograms of the opposite side of the chest. While some evidence suggests an increased risk of cancer in the other breast, the risk overall appears to be low.

It helps to know whether you have a genetic predisposition for breast cancer (genetic testing and counseling are recommended for all men with breast cancer). The American Society of Clinical Oncologists recommends opposite-breast screening if you carry a genetic variant linked to breast cancer.

the opposite, suggest cancer is there when none exists. Test results that are wrong or inconclusive can cause a lot of needless stress and anxiety and create the need for additional testing.

SUPPLEMENTAL SCREENING

If you have dense breast tissue or are at high risk of a second breast cancer — because of a genetic variant, for example — you may have additional options for screening, depending on:

- Your personal preferences, such as how comfortable you are with receiving a false-positive result, which occurs when imaging identifies a suspicious area that upon further testing is found to be benign.
- Practical matters, such as availability of tests near you and insurance coverage.

As you may already know, dense breast tissue can be difficult to screen for breast cancer. On a mammogram, dense breast tissue appears as a solid white area. This makes it difficult to see through and can mask the presence of a tumor.

There's evidence that supplemental tests, in addition to mammography, may help detect breast cancer in dense breast tissue. But it's not always clear who benefits from additional tests and how much of a benefit is gained. Additional tests carry additional risks, and no additional testing method has been proved to reduce the risk of dying of breast cancer.

If you — like almost half of women who have mammograms — have dense breast tissue, it's important to discuss supplemental screening with your oncologist or primary care doctor, taking into account your other risk factors, such as your family history, genetic profile, tumor biology, time since diagnosis, menopausal status and other factors. Tailoring surveillance to your individual experience is the best way to get the most out of screening.

Supplemental screening is also an option if you're considered at high risk for breast cancer. This might include having a genetic variant associated with breast cancer, being diagnosed before age 50, having an atypical form of breast cancer, or having breast cancer not detected on mammogram (also known as mammographically occult breast cancer). Insurance companies aren't always explicit about coverage for these tests, so it's a good idea to check with them directly before scheduling a test, to avoid surprises later.

Supplemental tests for breast cancer screening may include:

Breast MRI
A breast MRI uses magnetic resonance imaging along with an injected dye to scan your breasts and create detailed functional images of them — not just of their anatomy but also of blood vessel formation in the area. In breast cancer survivors who have dense breast tissue, a breast MRI is better able to detect breast cancer than a mammogram or ultrasound alone. For women with dense breasts and a breast cancer history, and for those diagnosed with breast cancer at age 50 or younger, annual MRI may be beneficial. In fact, the American College of Radiology recommends an MRI of the breasts once a year, in addition to annual mammograms, for women meeting these criteria.

Molecular breast imaging (MBI)
MBI is a supplemental imaging technique that uses a special camera (gamma camera) that records the activity of an injected radioactive tracer as it circulates in the body. Normal tissue and cancerous tissue react differently to the tracer, which can be seen in the images produced by the gamma camera. MBI can be used in some people as an alternative to MRI.

3-D mammogram (breast tomosynthesis)

Tomosynthesis uses X-rays to collect multiple images of the breast from several angles. The images are synthesized by a computer to form a 3-D image of the breast. This makes it easier to spot abnormalities in breast tissue. Using tomosynthesis reduces the rate of false positives compared with two-dimensional mammograms, especially in women under 50 with dense breasts. Many mammogram centers are transitioning to incorporate 3-D mammograms as part of the standard mammogram technology, regardless of breast density.

Contrast-enhanced imaging

Contrast-enhanced mammography (CEM) is a newer tool for detecting breast cancer. This test combines mammography with injection of a dye to provide contrast-enhanced images of the breasts. Studies are also being done to investigate the possibility of using contrast enhancement with other tests, such as ultrasound. Since it's so new as of this writing, it has limited

---

" I had a lumpectomy and when I do a self-breast exam, it is very hard to tell if what I am feeling is scar tissue or a new lump. I have gone to my provider a few times and it turns out to be nothing. I have rechecks every six months, and when the time for the appointment approaches, the anxiety increases. Antidepressants and antianxiety meds have helped me cope. It is hard to find the balance between 'getting on with life' and the fear of recurrence. — L.M.

availability for now. But the hope is that CEM will provide results similar to those of breast MRI but at a lower cost and with more potential uses, such as real-time guided biopsies.

DEALING WITH UNCERTAINTY

One of the most difficult aspects of follow-up care after primary breast cancer treatment is dealing with the uncertainty of whether or not the cancer will come back. Some people feel that testing will help them deal with this uncertainty. When asked, most say they want to be tested for a possible recurrence. And why not? Learning that your test results were normal can relieve a lot of anxiety and let you breathe a sigh of relief, at least until the next round of testing.

But testing has its pitfalls. Often tests will reveal a slight deviation or small abnormality that may need to be evaluated. And one test often leads to more tests, especially because very few tests are definitive enough to produce certain results by themselves.

It's also important to remember that just as tests can sometimes find more than you want them to, they can also miss things, such as a cancer recurrence. Negative results aren't a guarantee that no cancer is present.

Instead of focusing on things outside your control, you might choose to focus on those factors you do have some control over. This includes things like eating well, being physically active, getting enough rest and finding healthy ways to handle stress and anxiety.

Keep in mind that this is your life. You get to have a say in how much of your time and energy is taken up by testing and waiting for results. Have an honest discussion with your primary care doctor, your oncologist and

TREATING RECURRENT BREAST CANCER

Treatment options for recurrent breast cancer depend on several factors, including the extent of the disease, the time since treatment of the primary cancer, the type of treatment you received for your first breast cancer and the state of your overall health. Your doctor also considers your goals and your preferences for treatment.

Treatment for local or regional recurrence typically starts with surgery, if feasible, and may include radiation if you haven't had it before. Chemotherapy and endocrine therapy also may be recommended before or after surgery.

Many treatments exist for metastatic breast cancer. Your options will depend on the previously mentioned factors, the organs that are affected, and whether or not the cancer is causing symptoms. If one treatment doesn't work or stops working, you may be able to try other treatments. Read Chapter 5 for more on living with metastatic breast cancer.

other key members of your health care team. Let them know your preferences and values as well as your questions and concerns about your personal risk.

3

Staying healthy

Even after breast cancer treatment, it's important to continue taking good care of your body. The recommendations for cancer survivors are no different from those for anyone who wants improved health: Eat a balanced diet, exercise, maintain a healthy weight, get good sleep, avoid tobacco and alcohol or limit the amount of alcohol you drink.

In the short term, these healthy habits can make you feel better and more energized during your recovery. In the long term, positive lifestyle choices may influence positive health outcomes — possibly helping to reduce the chances of a breast cancer recurrence.

Another priority when it comes to your health is attending regular checkups with your primary care doctor in addition to visits with your oncology team.

Along with being monitored for signs of recurrence, it's important to undergo routine health screenings for other common conditions.

Juggling healthy habits along with all your other responsibilities may seem out of reach, but it doesn't have to be. This chapter provides tips and suggestions for how to tend to your health so that you can enjoy the years ahead.

FOLLOW A HEALTHY DIET

Eating nutritious foods can help you regain your strength, rebuild healthy tissue and feel good.

An eating plan that's rich in fruits, vegetables and whole grains is associated with longer life in breast cancer survivors. What's more, a healthy eating pattern may reduce your risk of other serious conditions, such as heart disease.

Focus on a colorful variety of plant-based foods that include whole grains and all types of legumes - beans, peas and lentils. Cook with healthy fats, such as olive oil. For more on healthy food choices, see pages 44-45.

What about supplements?

It's tempting to think that taking supplements might make you healthier, but the evidence for this is mixed at best. A small number of studies suggest that breast cancer survivors who take vitamin C and vitamin D after breast cancer treatment may increase their longevity. Multivitamins and vitamin E may have similar benefits. On the other hand, there's also good evidence that taking such antioxidant supplements, depending on the timing around treatment, can result in worse outcomes. More research is needed to clarify these findings.

WHAT TO EAT

To give your body the right kinds of fuel for cancer survival, go for variety — no one food contains all the nutrients you need, so aim to eat from all the food groups.

Go for	Go easy on
Plant-based foods — including all the suggestions below. Plant-based whole foods are rich in fiber, unlike animal-based foods. Aim for at least 30 grams of fiber every day. Research suggests fiber improves survival after a breast cancer diagnosis.	Animal-based foods, especially: • Red meat. • Processed meats, including hot dogs, deli meat, sausage and beef jerky.
A colorful variety of fruits and vegetables, such as: • Green grapes, kiwi fruit, broccoli, green beans, spinach and other dark leafy greens. • Red grapes, apples, strawberries, watermelon, red peppers and beets. • Blueberries, plums and eggplant. • Oranges, peaches, pineapple, carrots and sweet potatoes.	Foods and beverages containing added sugars or sweeteners, including: • Sweetened carbonated beverages, tea, coffee and energy drinks. • Sweet baked goods, such as cakes, cookies and pies. • Candy. • Sugary breakfast cereals.

Go for	Go easy on
Whole grains such as: • Brown rice. • Whole-wheat bread (try it sprouted). • Oil-free corn tortillas. • Whole-grain pasta. • Oatmeal. • Quinoa. • Popcorn. • Barley. • Bulgar.	Refined grains, such as those found in: • White bread and many "wheat" breads. • Many store-bought baked goods, pastas, and breakfast cereals.
Legumes, including: • Beans such as black, kidney, pinto, navy, black eyed-peas and others. • Lentils. • Lima beans. • Soy-based foods, such as tofu or tempeh.	Ultra-processed foods such as: • Chicken nuggets. • Frozen pizza and other ready-to-heat meals. • Instant soups. • Chips. • Snack cakes and packaged cookies.
Unsaturated fats, such those as found in: • Avocados. • Olive oil. • Nuts and seeds.	Saturated fats, such as those found in: • Animal-based foods including meat, cheese and eggs. • Coconut and coconut oil. • Palm oil and palm kernel oil. • Some fried and processed foods.

Supplements aren't intended to replace food. They can't replicate all the complex nutrients and interconnected benefits of whole foods, such as fruits and vegetables. For example, while you can get vitamin C from either an orange or a supplement, you won't get the fiber contained in the orange if you just take the supplement.

It's also important to know that more isn't better. In fact, large amounts of certain nutrients can hurt you. The rule of thumb is to take no more than 100% of the daily recommended intake of any nutrient. Before taking any new supplement, be sure to talk to your primary care doctor and oncology team, especially if you're still on medications related to your breast cancer treatment.

STRIVE FOR A HEALTHY WEIGHT

Mounting evidence indicates that sticking to a healthy weight may reduce your risk of breast cancer recurrence and secondary cancers, and help you live longer. Underweight, overweight and obesity are associated with an increased risk of recurrence among breast cancer survivors. Survivors who fall into these weight ranges may have a lower chance of survival due to breast cancer or other causes compared to those with a healthy weight. Gaining a large amount of weight may also increase your risks.

What is a healthy weight?
If you think you need to modify your weight, first determine what weight is appropriate for you. These three factors can help.
*   **Body mass index** (BMI) Your BMI considers your height and weight in determining whether you have a healthy or unhealthy percentage of body fat. A BMI of 18.5 to 24.9 is considered a healthy range.

WILL EATING SOY INCREASE MY RISK OF BREAST CANCER RECURRENCE?

It was once thought that soy foods increase the risk of breast cancer and breast cancer recurrence. However, current research doesn't bear this out. For example, one study compared breast cancer recurrence in U.S. and European populations compared with East Asian communities, which tend to consume higher amounts of soy-based foods. The risk of breast cancer recurrence among these populations is similar, suggesting that a moderate amount of soy doesn't increase the chances of recurrence. In fact, soy consumption may reduce breast cancer recurrence, making it a safe and healthy alternative to animal protein.

Soy supplements, on the other hand, generally contain higher levels of plant estrogens, called isoflavones. Some studies have suggested a link between these supplements and an increased risk of breast cancer in women who have a family or personal history of breast cancer. Cancer experts recommend avoiding these products.

Keep in mind that BMI is a good but imperfect guide. Muscle weighs more than fat, for instance, so if you're very muscular and physically fit, you can have a high BMI without added health risks.
- **Waist circumference** Waist circumference is a useful way to measure how much abdominal fat you

have. Too much abdominal fat is linked to a greater risk of heart disease and other related conditions, such as high blood pressure, high cholesterol and diabetes. A measurement exceeding 40 inches in men and 35 inches in women is associated with increased health risks.

- **Medical history** To get a more complete picture of your weight status, talk to your primary care doctor. Along with your BMI and waist circumference, a thorough evaluation of your medical history can help determine if you may benefit from losing some weight.

Set SMART goals

Achieving and maintaining a healthy weight is about making gradual, healthy changes in your diet and exercise habits. Over time, these habits help you achieve a healthy weight and they eventually become engrained in your lifestyle.

While that sounds simple, it can be difficult to put into practice. That's where SMART goals come in. SMART stands for specific, measurable, attainable, relevant and time-limited. Having SMART goals means starting off with small, reasonable goals and a concrete plan for how to achieve each of them.

- **Specific** State exactly what you want to achieve, how you're going to do it and when you want to achieve it. For example, instead of saying you'll improve your diet overall, aim to swap your afternoon sugary snack for a serving of fresh fruit. Instead of just saying you'll exercise more, set a goal of walking 15 minutes every morning.
- **Measurable** Track your progress by measuring it. Use an app, log or activity device to record the changes you're making to your diet and physical

activity. Recording your accomplishments can help you see your progress and keep you motivated.

- **Attainable** Set yourself up for success. Create a goal that's realistic and that you have enough time and resources to achieve. Setting small, short-term goals allows you to celebrate successes as you build toward a long-term goal.
- **Relevant** Set goals that are pleasing and meaningful to you and that fit where you're at in your life right now. In other words, if you really hate jogging, try hiking or swimming instead.
- **Time-limited** Pick a deadline for your goal that you can realistically meet and then strive to meet it.

Keep in mind that it takes time to form new habits, and you may experience some setbacks along the way. Many people do better when they have support from family and friends. Many enjoy the camaraderie of a fitness class. Discussing your weight goals with a registered dietitian or a certified fitness trainer may be helpful. Weight or exercise programs may help you stay on track.

STAY ACTIVE

Regular physical activity is probably the closest thing to an elixir of life that humans will ever encounter. Being active doesn't just help with weight loss and maintenance. It also reduces health risks — including the risk of cancer recurrence — and it improves long-term survival.

These benefits are reflected in medical research. For example, one critical analysis of 10 studies compared the activity levels of more than 23,000 women who had been diagnosed with breast cancer. Compared to the least active women, those who were highly active after diagnosis had a 40% lower rate of death due to breast cancer and a 42% lower rate of death due to any cause.

In the shorter-term, exercise is an important and proven way to increase your overall well-being and may speed your recovery after cancer treatment. Being physically active can help:

- Reduce side effects of cancer treatment, such as fatigue and insomnia.
- Increase your strength and endurance.
- Increase bone density.
- Boost your immune system.
- Lessen anxiety and depression.
- Improve your quality of life.

What's recommended?

The American Cancer Society recommends that cancer survivors avoid a sedentary lifestyle, returning to normal activities as soon as is reasonable. In other words, sit less and move more.

The chart on the next page provides physical activity guidelines for cancer survivors. Moderate activity includes walking briskly, dancing, canoeing, lawn mowing, or gardening — any activity where you're

---

“Physical exercise was always important to me but has become even more so since my diagnosis and as I age. Engaging in meaningful exercise provides me with a chance to release my thoughts and engage in an activity where I'm not always thinking about cancer. It has also allowed me the opportunity to socialize with others, which is so incredibly important to our emotional health and well-being. — L. K.

Weekly physical activity recommendations for cancer survivors
150–300 minutes of moderate aerobic activity
Or
75–150 minutes of vigorous aerobic activity
Or
A combination of moderate and vigorous activity
And
Strength training exercises for all major muscle groups at least two times a week

working hard but you can talk while you perform the exercise. Vigorous activity, such as jogging or running, fast biking, cross country skiing, or digging, uses greater effort, making it hard to get more than a couple of words out without a breath.

Getting started
Be sure to consider where you are in your recovery as well as your current health status. If you've been inactive for a long time or if you're starting a new exercise routine, get someone from your health care team to discuss your plans with you and OK them first.

Once it's safe to begin exercising, ease into it. If you do too much too soon, you could injure yourself or get discouraged. It's better to start slowly, gradually increasing your effort and your intensity level as your fitness level improves. Remember, set yourself up for success.

If you're new to exercise, think about the sorts of activities you might enjoy doing. Maybe it's walking, dancing or going to a yoga class with a friend. If you're not sure what you like, try different types of exercise. Don't force yourself to keep doing something you don't enjoy. The best kind of exercise is the kind you find pleasurable, you're willing to do and will want to continue doing.

PRIORITIZE GOOD SLEEP

Sleep is an important issue as a cancer survivor. Many people find that they feel tired and fatigued for several months or even years after they complete their cancer treatments. This lack of energy often stems from the physical and emotional impact of a cancer diagnosis and from the effects of cancer treatment. Sleep can help restore your energy.

Ironically, good sleep can be hard to come by after treatment. One study of 200 breast cancer survivors found that more than one-third experienced sleep difficulties. Problems included difficulty falling asleep, staying asleep, or waking too early.

If you're having sleep difficulties, know that sleep quality often improves the further out from treatment you are. Sometimes, work schedules, family responsibilities and other concerns make it difficult to get the rest you need. Do your best. Quality sleep can make the rest of life more doable. Here are some steps to get a more restful night's sleep.

Create a restful environment
Keep your room cool, dark and quiet. Exposure to light in the evenings might make it more challenging to fall asleep. Consider using room-darkening shades, ear-plugs, a fan or white noise to create a soothing environment.

Stick to a sleep schedule
Go to bed and get up at the same time every day, including weekends. Being consistent reinforces your body's sleep-wake cycle.

Unwind before bedtime
Avoid prolonged use of light-emitting digital screens — such as phones, tablets or TVs — just before bedtime. Doing calming activities before bedtime — such as taking a bath, reading a book or meditating — might promote better sleep.

Don't lie awake in bed
If you don't fall asleep within about 20 minutes of going to bed, leave your bedroom and do something relaxing. Read or listen to soothing music. Go back to bed when you're tired. Repeat as needed but continue to maintain your sleep schedule and wake-up time.

Limit daytime naps
Long daytime naps can interfere with nighttime sleep. Try to limit naps to no more than one hour and avoid napping late in the day.

Get moving
Regular physical activity can promote better sleep. But avoid being active too close to bedtime since activity can be stimulating in the short term.

Manage worries

Take time to wind down mentally and emotionally before bedtime. If your day has been crowded, stress management can help. Write down what's still on your mind and then set it aside for tomorrow. Start with the basics, such as getting organized, setting priorities and delegating tasks. Relaxation exercises, such as guided imagery or meditation, can help ease anxiety. Some people find it helpful to think about specific things they're grateful for at the end of the day.

Seek treatment

If you often have trouble sleeping, contact your primary care doctor. Identifying and treating any underlying causes of insomnia can help you get better sleep. To learn about recommended treatments for chronic sleep troubles, turn to page 64.

DON'T SMOKE OR VAPE

Breast cancer survivors who smoke or use other forms of tobacco are at greater risk of dying prematurely than people who don't use tobacco. One recent study looked at more than 54,000 women diagnosed with breast cancer who actively smoked, quit smoking or had never smoked. Those who actively smoked had a significantly higher rate of cancer-related death compared to women who had never smoked or quit smoking, and a higher rate of death due to any cause.

Quitting can substantially improve your odds of living longer. It's no wonder, then, that the American Cancer Society and the American Society of Clinical Oncology Breast Cancer recommend that breast cancer survivors who currently smoke quit smoking.

Get help quitting
If you've tried quitting without much success or want to quit but don't know where to begin, you aren't alone. It can be tough to stop smoking — especially without help. In fact, most people go through several attempts before successfully quitting. It may take more than one try, but you can do it.

A wealth of free information and advice is available to help you stop using tobacco. Trustworthy resources include the:
- American Cancer Society.
- Centers for Disease Control and Prevention (CDC).
- www.SmokeFree.gov hosted by the National Cancer Institute (NCI).

These organizations provide detailed information online. The CDC also offers free phone coaching. If you prefer text messaging, the National Cancer Institute offers messaging support through its SmokefreeTXT program, which you can find at www.SmokeFree.gov. There are also a variety of smart phone apps designed to help smokers quit.

Other valuable sources of support may include:
- Family.
- Friends.
- A member of your health care team.
- A counselor.
- A support group.

Consider quit-smoking products
Several quit-smoking products approved by the U.S. Food and Drug Administration (FDA) can greatly increase your chance of success. These products can help reduce nicotine cravings and withdrawal symptoms — making it more likely that you'll stop smoking for good. Some people turn to vaping as an

alternative to smoking. However, vaping is not a safe alternative to tobacco and research suggests it's bad for your heart and lungs.

Quit-smoking products fall into two main categories:

- **Nicotine replacement products** Options include patches, gum, lozenges, spray and inhaler. Although some are available without a prescription, it's best to talk with a member of your health care team before trying them.
- **Prescription medications** Bupropion and varenicline are two prescription medications that don't contain nicotine.

AVOID ALCOHOL

Investigation into the link between alcohol and cancer recurrence is ongoing. To date, it appears that avoiding alcohol may reduce the risk of cancer recurrence.

Research aimed specifically at breast cancer survivors has been somewhat inconsistent. Some studies have failed to show an association between alcohol consumption and breast cancer recurrence. However, many other studies suggest that consuming alcohol increases the risk of breast cancer recurrence or the risk of developing a second primary breast cancer. The risk may be particularly high for breast cancer survivors who are postmenopausal, obese, or who were diagnosed with estrogen receptor-positive tumors, but more research is needed.

The American Cancer Society recommends that people with a history of cancer avoid drinking any alcohol. If you choose to drink, remember these limits:

- No more than one drink a day for women.
- No more than two drinks a day for men.

One drink refers to a specific amount:
- Beer: 12 fluid ounces (355 milliliters).
- Wine: 5 fluid ounces (148 milliliters).
- Distilled spirits (80 proof): 1.5 fluid ounces (44 milliliters).

GET REGULAR HEALTH SCREENINGS

Follow-up cancer care may be foremost in your mind at medical visits, but don't overlook important preventive health screenings.

Cancer screenings

It's recommended that breast cancer survivors who do not have a hereditary breast cancer syndrome receive the same cancer screenings as the general public. These include:

- **Cervical cancer** If you have a cervix and are 21 to 29 years old, get screened every three years with a Pap test. If you have a cervix and are 30 to 65 years of age, get screened either every three years with a Pap test, every five years with a high-risk human papillomavirus (hrHPV) test, or every five years with both a Pap test and an hrHPV test.
- **Colorectal cancer** Colon cancer screenings are recommended between the ages of 45 and at least 75 for people who are at average risk of colorectal cancer. In some cases, screenings may be recommended up to age 85. Screenings may be done using colonoscopy, stool tests, flexible sigmoidoscopy or virtual colonoscopy, also known as CT colonography. How often you're screened depends on your risk level and the type of screening. Talk to your primary care team about the colorectal test that's best for you.

- **Lung cancer** Lung cancer screening is recommended if you currently smoke or have smoked within the past 15 years and you have a history of smoking 20 or more packs per year. The screening is a low-dose CT scan that's performed annually.

Routine health screenings

You should receive the same routine tests as the general population to regularly screen for:

- High blood pressure.
- Diabetes.
- High cholesterol.

Treatment-related screenings

Certain treatments for breast cancer may affect bone and heart health. Depending on your treatment regimen and other factors, a member of your health care team may monitor you for osteoporosis or heart disease.

Osteoporosis

Breast cancer and its treatment can affect bone cells, inhibiting bone formation or causing bone loss, which increases your risk of osteoporosis.

As a result, part of your follow-up care may involve monitoring for osteoporosis. Your primary care doctor may recommend a baseline dual-energy X-ray absorptiometry (DEXA) scan and then a repeat DEXA scan every one to two years thereafter if any of the following apply:

- You're postmenopausal.
- You take an aromatase inhibitor.
- You're premenopausal and taking tamoxifen, an endocrine-disrupting GnRH agonist or both.
- You develop premature menopause due to cancer treatment.

SHOULD MEN BEING TREATED WITH ADJUVANT ENDOCRINE THERAPY GET THEIR BONE DENSITY TESTED?

It's unclear how endocrine therapy affects bone density in male bodies. As a result, it's hard to say whether bone density testing is necessary. Mayo Clinic experts recommend:

- For men over 50, taking daily supplements of calcium (1,200 milligrams daily) and vitamin D3 (800 to 1,000 international units [IU]).
- Asking your health care team about using a fracture risk assessment tool (FRAX score) to help determine whether you need baseline and follow-up dual-energy X-ray absorptiometry (DEXA) testing during adjuvant endocrine therapy.

Cardiovascular disease

Some conventional chemotherapy drugs used to treat cancer can increase your risk of heart problems. Heart problems can also happen with newer targeted therapy drugs and with radiation therapy.

Whether you're at risk of heart problems after cancer treatment depends on how healthy your heart is and the specific drugs you received. Your risk may be higher if you have other risk factors for cardiovascular disease, including smoking, high blood pressure, diabetes, high cholesterol or obesity. You may be screened 6 to 12 months after breast cancer treatment if you were treated with any of these therapies:

- Anthracycline chemotherapy (most commonly doxorubicin).
- High-dose radiotherapy.
- Lower-dose radiotherapy in an area that included the heart.
- Trastuzumab, pertuzumab, or other HER2-directed therapy.

Screening may also be recommended if any of these factors apply to you:
- You were 60 or older at the time of cancer treatment.
- You experienced heart problems at any time before or during treatment, such as heart valve disease or heart attack.
- You currently have signs and symptoms of heart problems.

An echocardiogram is the gold standard tool used to screen for heart problems. It uses sound waves to produce images of your heart.

Oncologists and heart doctors, also called cardiologists, sometimes work together to provide care for people who have a risk of heart problems during and after cancer treatment. This area of medicine is sometimes referred to as cardio-oncology.

MAXIMIZE HEALTHY BENEFITS

After treatment, healthy habits have added benefits. They can improve your quality of life, lower the risk of the cancer coming back, and help you live longer.

4

Lingering or late side effects

Cancer treatment can save or extend lives. But it can also cause side effects, some of which can linger or appear long after treatment for early-stage breast cancer is over. And if you're undergoing additional treatment to reduce the chances of the cancer returning or to manage any leftover or remaining cancer, also called residual cancer, that treatment can also have side effects.

Symptoms such as pain, low mood, fatigue or hot flashes may linger or worsen over time. You may feel disappointed and discouraged that ongoing side effects are impacting your daily life. Or you may tell yourself, "It's a small price to pay for being alive. I'll manage."

You've made it this far and that's worth cheering. But if ongoing side effects are impacting your life, speak up. Talk to someone on your health care team. There may be treatments and strategies available to relieve your symptoms. This chapter is a good place to start learning about them. It covers a wide range of cancer-related side effects, along with research-based therapies and lifestyle interventions to treat them.

GENERAL SIDE EFFECTS

Each type of cancer treatment — surgery, radiation, drugs — affects the body differently, but certain side effects are common across treatments.

Fatigue

Ask people who've completed breast cancer treatment which side effect bothers them most, and many will say fatigue. It's common to experience some ongoing fatigue in the first months or even years after treatment. For a few people, the fatigue can be such that it gets in the way of everyday activities, including working and spending time with family and friends.

Cancer treatment and cancer itself can contribute to low energy. Fatigue can also be a reaction to the physical and emotional toll that cancer takes. Fortunately, in most cases, energy levels rebound over time.

How it's treated
If fatigue is keeping you from doing the things you enjoy, talk to your primary care doctor, who can check you for medical causes of your fatigue that may need to be treated. In addition, the following steps can help reduce or lessen fatigue.

Physical activity Research suggests that increased activity may be one of the best ways to reduce fatigue.

Exercising might sound like the last thing that you want to do when you're tired, so go slow. Make your goal to simply move more. Walk to the mailbox or to the end of the block and back. Gradually work your way up to 30 minutes of moderate exercise, such as brisk walking, bike riding or swimming — something that leaves you at least slightly breathless — five days a week. If you haven't been physically active lately, check with a member of your health care team before you begin a more vigorous activity routine to make sure it's safe.

Psychotherapy Negative thoughts and emotions can sap your energy and make you feel tired. Talking with a therapist may help you learn to replace overly negative thoughts with a more realistic or positive outlook.

Integrative therapies Some cancer survivors report that treatments such as acupuncture, massage and mindfulness training help to relieve symptoms of fatigue. Supplements that contain ginseng have been shown to relieve fatigue in small studies. If you're interested in trying supplements, discuss them with your health care team, as ginseng and other supplements can also present risks, such as interfering with certain medications.

Medications Medications may be available to treat the underlying cause of your fatigue. For instance, if you're depressed, there are medications that can help reduce the depression and improve your sense of well-being. If you're experiencing chronic pain, certain medications can be very helpful in managing the pain, which in turn can go a long way toward decreasing fatigue. But certain pain medications can make fatigue worse, so work with your health care team to achieve the proper balance.

> Be your own advocate. Ask questions if you do not understand. If a drug gives you side effects, speak up. Ask about options and alternatives. Do not let providers treat you like everyone else. You are an individual. — L. M.

Insomnia

Good sleep is a vital part of feeling better and more energetic. For some cancer survivors, that kind of restorative rest can be difficult to attain.

Insomnia is a common sleep problem that can make it hard to fall asleep, stay asleep or both. With insomnia, you might wake up feeling groggy and worn out. Insomnia can impact your energy level and mood, not to mention your work performance, quality of life and overall health. Many people struggle with poor sleep even before a cancer diagnosis.

Anxiety, depression, chronic pain and medically induced menopause symptoms, such as hot flashes, may affect how well you sleep, too.

How it's treated

A variety of therapies exist to help improve sleep. But first, one of the best things you can do to promote better sleep is to establish and maintain basic healthy sleep habits (see pages 52-53 for detailed tips). Having these habits in place will contribute to the success of other sleep therapies you might try.

Cognitive behavioral therapy for insomnia Cognitive behavioral therapy for insomnia (CBT-I) is the first line of treatment for most people with chronic insomnia. The therapy is a structured program that typically takes place over four to eight sessions and is led by a sleep specialist, though there are also mobile apps that help people engage in CBT-I on their own. If you choose to do CBT-I with a specialist, either in person or online, that person will teach you to recognize and change beliefs that affect your ability to sleep. You will also learn to develop good sleep habits and avoid behaviors that keep you from sleeping well.

Numerous studies have shown the effectiveness of CBT-I in relieving insomnia. Unlike pills, CBT-I addresses the underlying causes of insomnia rather than just relieving symptoms, making it more effective than medications in many cases.

Treating underlying problems If anxiety, depression, pain or hot flashes are affecting your sleep, treating those problems may help. See page 69 for more on treating anxiety and depression, page 79 for treating pain and page 84 for treating hot flashes.

Integrative therapies Acupuncture, massage and mindfulness exercises, such as meditation, may help to improve how well you sleep.

Medications Sleep medications are typically used for occasional insomnia caused by jet lag, for example. They're considered a treatment of last resort for chronic insomnia and not recommended for long-term use. In general, it's preferable to improve your sleep-related habits through lifestyle changes or CBT-I. Here are some temporary solutions a member of your health care team may recommend:

- **Over-the-counter sleep aids** Nonprescription sleep medications may contain antihistamines that can make you drowsy, but they're not intended for regular use. They can worsen symptoms of restless leg syndrome, a condition that makes you feel like you need to move your legs, which itself can interrupt your sleep. Talk to your primary care doctor before you take these, as antihistamines may cause other side effects that may be worse in older adults.

- **Supplements and botanicals** For a better night's sleep, some people turn to supplements, teas and extracts. While most of these products are considered safe, evidence of their effectiveness is limited. One of the most well-researched sleep-related supplements is melatonin. Studies suggest that melatonin may help you fall asleep faster, but it probably won't help you stay asleep. Before taking any new supplement, check with your health care team.

- **Prescription medications** Once in a while, a sleeping pill prescribed on a short-term basis may help you through an especially rocky period. However, prescription sleep medications aren't recommended for long-term or regular use because of their side effects. In fact, when used regularly, many of these medicines make it *harder* for you to fall asleep naturally.

Changes in weight and appetite

Cancer treatment often impacts body weight. In some cases, it can cause unwanted weight gain. Or it can cause you to lose weight by suppressing your appetite. Stress, anxiety or depression also can change what you want to eat.

What you can do

Talk to your primary care doctor or a nutritionist about concerns you may have about your body weight. These professionals can help you establish goals and strategies to get you to a healthy weight. The following tips may also be helpful.

If you're aiming to gain weight:

- **Focus on your favorite foods** To jump-start your appetite, choose foods you really enjoyed before treatment.
- **Eat small meals throughout the day** You might find this works better than limiting yourself to traditional mealtimes.
- **Stay active** Physical activity, such as a short walk before a meal, can help you feel hungry.
- **Build muscle** If part of your weight loss includes loss of muscle, strength-training exercises can help you build your muscles back up.

If you're trying to lose weight:

- **Be patient with yourself** It can take time to shed the pounds gained during treatment. Aim for gradual weight loss, such as 2 pounds a month — which translates to 24 pounds a year, a substantial amount of weight loss.
- **Focus on healthy habits** Try incorporating exercise into your routine and eating a healthy diet. These habits may have the added benefit of reducing the chance of cancer recurrence. Chapter 2 has specific recommendations about physical activity and diet to promote health after cancer treatment.
- **Don't go it alone** While the advice to move more and eat healthfully may sound simple, it can be challenging to put into action — especially if these are new habits. You don't have to do it alone. Talk to a member of your health care team or a nutritionist. Enlist the support of family and friends. Consider enrolling in a weight or exercise program.

Cognitive changes

Do you ever feel like your mind isn't working as well as it did before cancer? It might not be your imagination. Some breast cancer survivors report post-treatment problems with memory, concentration or slow thinking. They report having a harder time learning new things, multitasking or remembering common words. The problem is sometimes called "brain fog" or "chemo brain," although cognitive changes may also result from the stress of diagnosis, cancer-related surgery or a variety of cancer treatments other than chemotherapy. Fatigue, insomnia, pain and depression all tend to make the problem worse.

What you can do
Talk to your primary care doctor if you're concerned about cognitive changes you're experiencing. You may be evaluated for underlying causes of your symptoms. In many cases, cognitive side effects improve on their own over time. But there are simple steps you can take to reduce mental fogginess and sharpen your mind.

Move your body Aerobic exercise, such as walking, hiking and other physical activities help boost your brain function.

Get organized Stay on track with physical or digital planners, sticky note reminders or digital reminders on your phone. Plan ahead by scheduling challenging tasks at the time of day when you have the most energy and mental focus.

Give your brain a workout Use your mind by doing brain puzzles, playing word games, taking a class or learning a new language.

WHAT IS INTEGRATIVE MEDICINE?

Integrative medicine refers to health care practices that traditionally haven't been part of conventional medicine. In many cases, as evidence of safety and effectiveness grows, these therapies are being combined with conventional medicine. If you want to learn more, turn to Chapter 8, which covers a variety of integrative treatment approaches.

Explore integrative therapies Integrative approaches, such as meditation and other mindfulness-based strategies, may improve your cognition. See Chapter 8 for more on integrative therapies.

Ask about cognitive rehabilitation therapy This option is available at some institutions, including Mayo Clinic. Cognitive rehabilitation therapists work with you to improve your thinking skills and maximize your success in your personal and work life.

Anxiety and depression

Many people experience feelings of sadness, anger or fear of cancer recurrence in the weeks and months after completing cancer treatment. Often those feelings lessen with time. But sometimes they deepen, developing into anxiety, depression or a combination of the two.

If your mental health is impairing your enjoyment of life or your ability to function, reach out to your primary care doctor or a mental health professional to get help. The support of family, friends and faith can also be very helpful.

> **❝** I've been able to cope with emotional ups and downs by relying on my faith and the power of prayer. I've also found it incredibly helpful to find a good psychologist or counselor that I felt comfortable enough with to discuss the roller coaster of emotions we all experience when receiving a cancer diagnosis. — L. K.

How it's treated

Depending on the severity of your symptoms, you might benefit from one or more of these options.

Self-care Make your mental health a priority by taking care of the basics — exercise, engage in healthy eating habits, and get enough sleep. Spend time with family and friends. These simple strategies can be powerful mood boosters.

Psychotherapy Sometimes called talk therapy, psycho-therapy can be an effective treatment for anxiety and depression. Cognitive behavioral therapy and mindfulness-based approaches are two options that may improve your symptoms. If possible, choose a therapist who has experience working with cancer survivors. Your cancer care team may be able to provide you with a recommendation.

Medications If your symptoms persist, your doctor may prescribe antidepressants or other medications to relieve symptoms, often in conjunction with psychotherapy.

WARNING SIGNS OF DEPRESSION

You may have depression if you have some or all these signs and symptoms most of the day, nearly every day:

- Feelings of sadness, tearfulness, emptiness or hopelessness.
- Angry outbursts, irritability or frustration, even over small things.
- Loss of interest or pleasure in most or all normal activities.
- Sleep disturbances, including insomnia or sleeping too much.
- Tiredness and lack of energy.
- Reduced appetite and weight loss or increased cravings for food and weight gain.
- Anxiety, agitation or restlessness.
- Slowed thinking, speaking or body movements.
- Feelings of worthlessness or guilt, fixating on past failures or self-blame.
- Trouble thinking, concentrating, making decisions and remembering things.
- Frequent or recurrent thoughts of death, suicidal thoughts, or suicide attempts.
- Unexplained physical problems, such as stomach pain or headaches.

WARNING SIGNS OF ANXIETY

Common anxiety signs and symptoms include:
- Excessive worry occurring more days than not for at least six months.
- Racing thoughts.
- Feelings of restlessness.
- Fatigue.
- Difficulty concentrating.
- Irritability.
- Muscle tension.
- Sleep disturbances, difficulty falling or staying asleep.
- Distress or inability to function in work or social settings.
- Physical problems such as shakiness, increased heart rate, tightness in the chest or rapid breathing.

SIDES EFFECTS OF LOCAL OR REGIONAL TREATMENTS

Cancer therapies such as surgery and radiation therapy treat a specific location or region of the body. These treatments may lead to certain longer-term side effects.

Scarring

All operations leave a physical scar. Some cancer survivors view their scars with pride — signs of a battle they fought and won. But scars can also be unwanted reminders of a difficult time, and they can affect how you feel about your body. Occasionally, scars can restrict movement and interfere with daily activities.

How it's treated
Most scars fade over time on their own. But you can also take steps to reduce their appearance.

Lifestyle measures These simple steps may help to minimize scarring:
- Following post-surgery instructions for proper wound care.
- Keeping the wound moist by applying a thin layer of petroleum jelly.
- Gently massaging scars (after getting approval from your surgeon).
- Protecting scars from sun exposure after surgery by covering them with clothing or applying sunscreen.
- Wearing a support bra.

Medical treatments Occasionally a scar might not fade or may continue to be uncomfortable after it's healed. Rarely, one or more of these treatments may be recommended to treat certain types of scars:
- Corticosteroid cream to ease itching.
- Silicone gel to flatten a scar.
- Injections of cortisone or other steroids to reduce scar thickness.
- Freezing a scar with liquid nitrogen (cryotherapy) to reduce or remove the scar.
- Laser treatments to flatten a scar.
- Low-level radiation therapy to shrink or remove a scar.
- Surgery to remove a scar and try to make the new scar look better.

Some of these treatments come with side effects of their own or may be less successful than you'd like. Be sure to

> After my mastectomies, I 'went flat.' I even like being flat. No bra, no prostheses, and no problems with clothing. I do not feel self-conscious any longer, though I did the first summer. The scars still burn a little in salt water or hot weather, but a flat chest is a welcome bargain for possible health. I do not have a partner, and understand that those who do may experience more emotions going flat. — P. W.

---

talk to your doctor or surgeon to determine whether a particular treatment will be beneficial for you.

Lymphedema

Lymphedema is swelling caused by a buildup of protein-rich fluid that usually drains through your body's lymphatic system. Surgery or radiation therapy that involves your lymph nodes can sometimes lead to lymphedema. The swelling typically develops in the arm on the side of your body that was treated for breast cancer. The wrist or hand may also be affected. In addition, swelling can develop in the treated chest and breast area.

Along with swelling, you may experience other symptoms of lymphedema, such as difficulty with movement or flexibility in the shoulder or arm. A hardening and thickening of the skin can also develop. The symptoms of lymphedema can cause discomfort, impact activities and affect your feelings about your appearance.

If you had breast surgery, you may have had some mild immediate swelling right after the surgery. This typically goes away in the first few weeks. If the swelling persists in your arm, hand or breast area, you may have lymphedema. Another sign of the condition can be new symptoms that develop weeks or years after surgery or radiation therapy, on the side of the body where the treatment occurred.

Most breast cancer survivors who develop lymphedema will do so in the first three years after surgery or radiation. Exercise seems to help prevent lymphedema, so don't be afraid to engage in strength training or aerobic exercise, or in active hobbies like gardening, woodworking or riding horses. There is no reliable evidence to support restricting physical activity to reduce the risk of lymphedema.

It's good to know the early warning signs of lymphedema, which often develop before swelling occurs. Early symptoms include:

- Aching.
- Tingling.
- Numbness.
- A sensation of fullness or heaviness.

Contact your cancer care team or primary care doctor if you notice any of these symptoms so that you can be evaluated for lymphedema. Early intervention is key. It's easier to control lymphedema if the condition is managed early. By being proactive, you'll be better able to maintain all the activities you enjoy. If symptoms are ignored, the condition can get worse and be harder to control.

How it's treated

There isn't a medication known to effectively treat lymphedema, but there are things you can do to reduce the severity and continue to enjoy an active lifestyle.

At-home techniques If you've already developed lymphedema, try these suggestions:

- **Physical activity** Exercises such as aerobic activity and strength training may help to reduce the symptoms of lymphedema. Staying active can allow you to continue your favorite activities.
- **Compression** Wearing a compression bandage, sleeve or bra may encourage trapped lymph fluid to flow and minimize swelling.
- **Moisturizing** Use moisturizing cream, especially in the winter, to keep the skin from drying out and forming cracks.
- **Injury avoidance** Fingers and hands are prone to small cuts and scrapes that are often ignored. If you have lymphedema, these small breaks in the skin can be vulnerable to infections. Cuts, scrapes and burns to your affected arm can also invite infection. Protect yourself from sharp objects. For example, shave with an electric razor or wear gloves when you do activities that could cause small cuts such as gardening or carpentry.
- **Loose clothing** To limit swelling, avoid wearing jewelry or clothing that restricts your affected arm or hand.

Therapy Your primary care doctor or a specialized lymphedema therapist may recommend techniques to reduce swelling. Common recommendations include:

- **Lymphatic massage** A lymphedema therapist may use a massage-like technique to move the fluid trapped in the swollen area toward an area with working lymph vessels. This process stimulates alternative routes for the fluid to drain.
- **Exercises** A lymphedema therapist may recommend specific exercises to help move the excess fluid out of a swollen area and increase your range of motion.

- **Pressure device** Your therapist may also recommend wearing a prescribed intermittent pressure device around your arm that inflates and deflates, moving lymph fluid up your arm and away from the fingers.

Surgical treatment If at-home and therapeutic treatments aren't effective, surgery may be considered. Surgery may also be an option for severe lymphedema. Procedures are available to:
- Transplant lymph nodes from a healthy area of the body to the affected arm.
- Create new paths in the lymph network to drain trapped fluid.
- Remove hardened tissue to improve the arm's function.

Restricted shoulder and arm movement
Tightness and pain in the shoulder and arm are common side effects immediately after breast cancer surgery. Radiation therapy can also cause this problem and contribute to reduced range of motion. The goal of recovery is to return to your full range of motion and activities.

Within six weeks of surgery, many people can raise both arms straight up over their head. Occasionally problems with range of motion last longer. For some people, the arm and shoulder stiffness doesn't develop until 3 to 12 months after surgery. This may be more likely if you've also undergone radiation therapy, especially if your range of motion was already limited before treatment. Lack of movement in the arm and shoulder after surgery can also increase your risk.

RISK OF INFECTION WITH LYMPHEDEMA

Lymph node surgery doesn't affect your overall immune function and ability to fight infections, even if you develop lymphedema. However, your risk of infection in the area affected by lymphedema can increase. If you've had prior infections in that part of your body, your doctor may prescribe antibiotics for you to keep on hand. That way, you can start taking them immediately once symptoms of infection appear.

What you can do

If you had breast cancer surgery, talk to your surgeon or cancer care team about what activities you should do and when you can start. Your health care team may recommend gentle arm and shoulder exercises to begin shortly after surgery. These exercises are designed to increase your range of motion and help maintain your arm function. You may also be encouraged to continue exercises during and after radiation therapy.

Arm and shoulder exercises can help you return to your regular activities more quickly. This period of healing may take time, so go slow and continue to increase your activity as your body allows. Ideally you will be able to return to all the activities you enjoyed prior to surgery and hopefully pick up some new hobbies.

If pain and stiffness continue to impact your life, talk with a member of your health care team. You may be referred to a physical or occupational therapist to help you restore range of motion and flexibility.

Discomfort and pain in the treated breast area
Pain is often unavoidable when you've had surgery. It's usually short-term and goes away on its own. For some breast cancer survivors, low-level pain or discomfort in the treated area continues for months after surgery.

Breast cancer surgery requires that some nerves in the breast be cut. Rarely, this can lead to persistent pain or discomfort in the in the chest wall, armpit or arm. This condition is called post-mastectomy pain syndrome. The most common side effects are:
- Burning sensations, shooting pain that comes and goes.
- Tingling or a pins-and-needles sensation.
- Loss of feeling or numbness.

How it's treated
You don't have to live with post-mastectomy pain or discomfort. Treatments are available to reduce or relieve your symptoms.

Physical therapy Increasing activity and range of motion, often under a physical therapist's direction, can alleviate many of these symptoms and help you return to the activities you enjoy.

Acupuncture, massage therapy and biofeedback
These techniques can be helpful, usually alongside physical therapy.

Medications Over-the-counter pain relievers may effectively reduce mild symptoms. For more severe pain, prescription medications such as antidepressants and antiseizure drugs may reduce your discomfort. Prescription painkillers such as opioids generally aren't recommended to treat pain that has become chronic.

Topical treatments Some creams and gels contain medicine that may help control pain, such as capsaicin.

Non-surgical procedures Certain types of pain, such as nerve pain or highly tender spots (trigger points) in the treated area, may improve with nonsurgical procedures. Your health care team may recommend injections of medicines that block pain. Radiofrequency ablation may be another option. This procedure uses heat generated by radio waves to target specific nerves and temporarily turn off their ability to send pain signals.

Surgery A doctor may recommend surgery to remove painful nerve tissue growth or to repair a painful surgical scar.

SIDE EFFECTS OF SYSTEMIC TREATMENTS

Systemic treatments are drugs that are taken orally or intravenously to treat cancer. They travel through the bloodstream, moving throughout your body. Chemotherapy, endocrine therapy, HER2-targeted therapies and immunotherapy are examples of systemic treatment, and they come with their own side effects.

Neuropathy
Some chemotherapy medications such as paclitaxel, docetaxel and carboplatin, can cause nerve damage, also called neuropathy. Neuropathy from chemotherapy often results in numbness and pain, usually in the hands and feet. People generally describe the pain as stabbing, burning or tingling.

PHANTOM BREAST PAIN

Some breast cancer survivors experience sensations that feel like they're happening to the removed breast. This is known as phantom breast syndrome. Common sensations include:
- Pain.
- Throbbing.
- Pressure.
- Tingling.
- Itching.

Treatment usually begins with temporary medications to reduce phantom pain. Your provider may then add noninvasive therapies, such as acupuncture and psychotherapy. More-invasive options include injections or implanted devices. Surgery is done only as a last resort.

How it's treated

Treatment is aimed at relieving the symptoms of neuropathy. Your health care team may recommend one or more of these options:

Home remedies To manage peripheral neuropathy and reduce pain:
- **Take care of your feet** Check regularly for blisters, cuts or calluses. Wear soft, loose cotton socks and padded shoes.
- **Exercise regularly** This can be as simple as walking three times a week.

WHEN BREAST SURGERY DOESN'T GO AS PLANNED

Most women who undergo breast reconstruction or breast-conserving surgery are happy with the results. But occasionally the surgery leads to:

- Problems with an implant, such as rupture, leakage or deflation.
- Scar tissue that forms and compresses the implant and breast tissue into a hard, unnatural shape.
- Death of all or a portion of a tissue flap, skin or fat due to a lack of blood supply.
- Very low risk of a rare cancer associated with breast implants.

Contact your surgeon if you're experiencing any problems related to your surgery. Correcting these complications may require additional surgery.

- **Quit smoking** Cigarette smoking can affect circulation, increasing the risk of foot problems and other neuropathy complications.
- **Eat healthy meals** This ensures that you get essential vitamins and minerals. Include fruits, vegetables, whole grains and lean protein in your diet.
- **Avoid excessive alcohol** It can worsen peripheral neuropathy.

Integrative therapies Certain complementary approaches, including acupuncture, might be helpful for neuropathy. Consult with your care team before trying any integrative treatment.

Medications Depending on the severity of your pain, your doctor may treat your pain with medication. Duloxetine is an antidepressant that has been proven to help some patients with neuropathy.

Muscle and joint pain
Certain types of chemotherapy, endocrine therapy and immunotherapy can cause soreness in the muscles or joints. The pain often subsides once treatment has ended. In some cases, the pain is longer lasting, or it develops months or years after treatment.

Muscle pain is sometimes accompanied by muscle weakness and cramps. If you have joint pain, your joints may feel swollen, tender or warm to the touch. The pain or discomfort may worsen when you're at rest and improve once you get moving.

" Breast cancer has left me with some neuropathy, osteoporosis, and the everpresent hot flashes, a little bit of heart valve damage, and some discomfort in the breasts. I look for ways to accommodate for these challenges and not let them slow me down. I wear cotton bras that irritate less, and ice my feet at night. I rest if I feel out of breath and have stopped training young horses so as to minimize the risk of broken bones. I definitely feel like I have become more accepting of these challenges as time goes by. — C.

How it's treated
Treatment for muscle or joint pain may depend on the severity of the discomfort. Self-care at home is often a good place to start.

Self-care For mild pain, your provider may recommend these at-home strategies:
- Over-the-counter pain relievers.
- Ice packs.
- Heating pads or warm baths.
- Massage.

Physical therapy Physical therapy can be helpful for some types of muscle or joint pain. Exercises can gently stretch and strengthen muscles and joints to improve symptoms.

Integrative therapies Certain treatments, such as acupuncture or therapeutic massage, may relieve your pain.

Medications If your pain is more persistent or severe, your provider may recommend:
- Steroid medicines, also called corticosteroids.
- Antidepressants or anti-seizure medications.
- Muscle relaxants.

Menopausal symptoms and sexual changes
If you're premenopausal, chemotherapy can cause your periods to stop and result in menopausal symptoms. Whether you're premenopausal or postmenopausal, endocrine therapy can lead to menopausal symptoms because the treatment either blocks female hormone receptors or reduces the amount of hormones your body makes. Symptoms may include:

I CAN'T TOLERATE THE SIDE EFFECTS OF ENDOCRINE THERAPY. WHAT SHOULD I DO?

Adjuvant endocrine therapy is recommended for 5 to 10 years for most people with hormone receptor-positive breast cancers because it can reduce the risk that cancer will recur in the breast or elsewhere in the body. But for some people, the side effects of endocrine therapy can make it hard to imagine taking the medication for years.

Adjuvant endocrine therapy does help decrease the risk of breast cancer recurrence. If you're experiencing significant side effects, talk to your cancer care team. Many symptoms can be managed by adjusting or changing the medication, or adding supportive therapies.

- Irregular periods or no periods.
- Hot flashes.
- Problems with your vagina, such as vaginal dryness that causes burning or itching, or pain during intercourse.
- Problems holding your urine or urinary tract problems.
- Fatigue and sleep problems.
- Memory and other problems, such as depression, mood swings and irritability.
- Other changes in your body, such as less muscle and more fat around your body, or thinning and loss of elasticity of your skin.
- Less interest in and enjoyment of sex (see Chapter 9 for more information).

> Hard menopause at 38 was a novel idea I could have done without. I watched myself grow old pretty fast. I mostly just don't notice anymore. Physical looks have never been too important to me. At first I felt a little betrayed by my body, but I did make peace with it. Learning to focus on the moment and not the future has been an asset to me in this journey. — C.

Over time, some women who were premenopausal at the time of their cancer diagnosis will start getting their periods again, but others will not. Generally, women in their late 40s or early 50s are more likely to experience permanent menopause due to cancer treatments than younger women.

How it's treated
Treatment focuses on relieving the signs and symptoms of menopause that are bothersome.

Self-care Some people find relief using these lifestyle strategies:
- **Layers** Dress in layers that you can easily remove. When a hot flash strikes, drink a cold glass of water, put a cool towel on your neck, or go somewhere cooler.
- **Pinpoint your triggers** Hot flashes may be triggered by hot beverages, caffeine, spicy foods, alcohol, stress, hot weather or even a warm room.
- **Practice relaxation techniques** Deep breathing, guided imagery, massage and progressive muscle relaxation may help with menopausal symptoms.
- **Exercise regularly** Get regular physical activity or exercise on most days.

CHANGES IN MALE BODIES

Because so many male breast cancers are hormone receptor positive, endocrine therapy is often recommended to reduce the risk of recurrence or control metastatic disease. As in women, endocrine therapy can cause side effects in men, too. Although not as well-studied as in women, small studies suggest that side effects in men may include:

- Changes in libido.
- Difficulty having or keeping an erection.
- Hot flashes.
- Mood swings.
- Blood clots.

Many of the remedies described in this chapter apply to men as well as women. For example, exercise can help you increase your energy level, maintain muscle strength and manage stress.

If you're experiencing hot flashes, which are common among people taking endocrine therapy, ask your primary care doctor or oncologist about potential treatments. Venlafaxine, an antidepressant, has been helpful for treating hot flashes in men with prostate cancer who are taking endocrine therapy.

If you're experiencing symptoms of sexual dysfunction, be sure to talk to your care team about specific therapies that might help. Speaking with a counselor or sexual health professional, alone or with your partner, is also recommended. But don't take testosterone or androgen supplements, as these might increase the level of estrogen in your body and thus increase your risk of breast cancer tumor growth.

Nonhormone medications These oral medications
have shown some benefits in decreasing hot flashes:
- Low-dose antidepressants, such as venlafaxine.
- Gabapentin, an anti-seizure medication.
- Clonidine, a pill or patch typically used to treat high
  blood pressure.
- Oxybutynin, a treatment for overactive bladder.

Nonhormone vaginal lubricants Over-the-counter,
water-based vaginal lubricants or silicone-based
lubricants may relieve discomfort from vaginal dryness.
For more detailed information about vaginal lubricants
and other ways to manage pain during sex due to
vaginal dryness, see page 134.

CAN I TAKE HORMONE THERAPY FOR MENOPAUSAL SYMPTOMS?

Menopausal hormone therapy taken orally or through the skin (transdermal) is an effective treatment for menopausal symptoms such as hot flashes and night sweats. These medications contain female hormones and are taken to replace just enough of the estrogen that the body stops making during menopause to reduce symptoms.

Hormone therapy used for breast cancer, also known as adjuvant endocrine therapy, does not contain female hormones. Adjuvant endocrine therapy works to change hormone levels in the body to deprive hormonally sensitive tumors of fuel they use to grow.

Current research suggests that certain types of menopausal hormone therapy may increase the risk of developing breast cancer. Menopausal hormone therapy may also increase the risk of recurrence for women with hormone-receptor positive breast cancer.

Before considering menopausal hormone therapy, talk to your cancer care team to determine if it's a safe option for you. The same holds true if you're considering vaginal hormones or birth control that contains estrogen, progesterone, or a combination of the two.

5

Living with metastatic breast cancer

When breast cancer spreads to other areas outside of the breast, such as bones, lungs or liver, it's referred to as metastatic breast cancer. Other terms commonly used are *advanced cancer* or *stage IV cancer*. Some people have metastatic breast cancer when they're first diagnosed, but metastases more often develop some time after treatment for a previous diagnosis of earlier stage breast cancer, when that treatment was unable to eradicate all the cancer cells. When cancer returns after an original diagnosis, it is referred to as a *recurrence*.

The process of diagnosis and treatment of recurrent breast cancer has some similarities to the first experience, but there are some key differences. If your oncologist suspects you may have recurrent breast cancer based on results of a mammogram or physical exam, or because of signs and symptoms, the oncologist may recommend additional tests to confirm the diagnosis.

Imaging tests may include magnetic resonance imaging (MRI), computerized tomography (CT), X-ray, bone scan or positron emission tomography (PET). Not every person needs every test. Your oncologist will determine which tests are most helpful in your situation. These tests can help determine whether a biopsy — a procedure to collect a tissue sample for lab testing — is needed to confirm whether cancer has spread to a specific area.

From the biopsy sample, a pathologist can determine if the cancer is a recurrence of cancer or a new type of cancer. Tests also show whether the cancer is sensitive to hormone treatment or targeted therapy since these may have changed since your original cancer diagnosis.

When cancer has spread to other organs, it is typically incurable. Nonetheless, treatment can help control the cancer effectively, with the goals of extending your life and helping you to live as well as possible, for as long as possible. As breast cancer treatments become more and more effective, people are surviving longer with metastatic breast cancer. Importantly, treatment can also relieve many symptoms that are caused by the cancer, improving quality of life in addition to length.

TREATMENT FOR METASTATIC BREAST CANCER

Whether you're newly diagnosed with metastatic breast cancer or have been previously treated for a breast cancer that has now recurred or progressed to an advanced stage, treatment of your metastatic breast cancer will likely be very different from that of early-stage breast cancer.

The goals of your treatment options will depend on your situation — such as the characteristics of the tumor, how long you've been without cancer, where and how far the cancer has spread, and whether the cancer is causing any symptoms or difficulties with specific organ functions.

Most importantly, treatment goals will depend on your preferences. When deciding on treatment options, it is important to discuss and consider not only the potential benefits of the treatment, but also the potential side effects. As a wider variety of treatment options becomes available, your providers may be able to select treatments that have a side effect profile you're willing to consider.

Treatment options

Depending on the characteristics of your breast cancer, treatments may include:

- **Endocrine therapy** If your cancer contains hormone receptors — which means that the breast cancer cells are dependent on female hormones to grow and multiply — you may benefit from a hormone treatment known as endocrine therapy. This treatment targets the estrogen receptor and blocks the tumor's access to estrogen, which in turn decreases cancer cell growth. In cancers that are dependent on estrogen, endocrine therapy is typically more effective than chemotherapy, particularly in the initial phases of the disease. In general, endocrine therapy also has fewer side effects than chemotherapy and can be more convenient, as there are several oral options.

- **Chemotherapy** Chemotherapy involves medications that kill rapidly growing cells. Because cancer cells typically replicate at a faster rate than healthy cells, chemotherapy can effectively kill cancer cells, regardless of whether they are dependent on estrogen or not. Your oncologist may recommend chemotherapy if your cancer is hormone receptor negative, if endocrine therapy is no longer working, or if your tumor has certain genetic alterations such as being HER2 positive.
- **Targeted therapy** This involves medications that interfere with specific cellular processes that allow cancer cells to grow more rapidly or become resistant to other treatments. Examples of targeted therapies include CDK 4/6 inhibitors, PI3 Kinase/AKT/mTOR pathway inhibitors, or HER2 directed therapy. Targeted therapies are often given in combination with other treatments such as endocrine therapy or chemotherapy.
- **Immunotherapy** Immunotherapy involves medications that stimulate your immune system to help it recognize and attack cancer cells. Cancer cells often produce proteins that help them hide from immune system cells. Immunotherapy works by interfering with that process. It might be an option in combination with chemotherapy if you have triple-negative breast cancer, which means that the cancer cells don't have receptors for estrogen, progesterone or HER2.
- **Clinical trials** Your oncologist may recommend a clinical trial that is appropriate for your circumstances. When you talk to your health care team about treatment options for metastatic breast cancer, ask if you qualify for a clinical trial. This question is an important way to advocate for

yourself and make sure you're getting the best possible care. Feel free to bring up participation in a clinical trial with your cancer care team if you are interested learning more about it. See Chapter 7 for more on clinical trials.

- **Supportive care treatments** Radiation therapy and surgery may be used in certain situations to ease symptoms caused by advanced breast cancer, such as pain, but these treatments typically aren't used to try to get rid of the cancer. Additionally, if cancer has spread to your bones, your doctor may recommend a bone-building drug to reduce your risk of developing broken bones or reduce bone pain you may experience.

After starting treatment, you'll have regular checkups to make sure that you're feeling well, your cancer symptoms are manageable and treatment side effects are tolerable. You'll also have regular blood tests and scans to ensure that the treatment is working and not causing problems in other organs. If your treatments aren't working or the side effects are not tolerated, your oncologist may recommend a different treatment.

Treatment goals
When considering your treatment plan, your oncologist is likely to have these goals for you in mind:
- The fewest side effects from the cancer for as long as possible.
- The fewest side effects from the treatment for as long as possible.
- The longest life.
- The best quality of life.

It's also important for you to think about your own priorities. Understanding what you want out of treatment can help guide your treatment decisions. Some people want to treat their cancer for as long as they can and are willing to undergo some discomfort to do so. Others would like to focus on quality of life rather than length of life, preferring to avoid harsh treatment side effects. It is critical to discuss your treatment goals with your cancer care team and your loved ones. Honest and frank communication can help make sure that everyone is on the same page and striving for the same goals.

YOUR EMOTIONS (AND HOW TO COPE)

Shock. Anger. Fear. Grief. These are all natural feelings after learning that you have metastatic breast cancer, yet coping with these strong emotions can be one of the biggest challenges you'll face. It's tempting to want to hide away or deny all that's happening. And there may be days when you do just that. But it may help to know that many people diagnosed with metastatic breast are able to continue living meaningful and fulfilling lives despite the challenges and uncertainties.

Here are some common feelings that people with metastatic breast cancer report having.

Anger
You're upset that you have to go through treatment again. Perhaps you find yourself lashing out at those around you or becoming furious with things that wouldn't have bothered you before. If you're religious, you may question how a benevolent, all-powerful being could allow this to happen to you.

Anger is an important stage of grief. Give yourself some freedom to express it. Unprocessed or suppressed,

GETTING A SECOND OPINION

If you've been diagnosed with metastatic breast cancer, a second opinion can help make sure your treatment plan is the best option for your cancer.

Here are questions to ask when you're getting a second opinion:

- Am I receiving the best and most up-to-date treatment for my type of breast cancer?
- Do I need a biopsy or any other tests that would provide more information about my cancer's characteristics?
- Are there any clinical trials that I am eligible for either now or in the future?
- How often should I have restaging scans?

Keep in mind that the team seeing you for the second opinion may recommend the same treatment plan as your primary team. This can give you peace of mind. A second opinion also may provide more details about your breast cancer and other treatments for you to consider. Often, it is safe to take some time to reflect on the options your team has discussed with you and make decisions aligned with your goals.

It's important that you know that it's OK to seek a second opinion. An experienced oncologist will not be offended if you say you'd like another perspective and, in fact, may welcome another point of view. You can ask your current oncologist or someone on your cancer care team, such as a patient navigator or social worker, for a referral, or you might get a recommendation from family, friends, or your primary care doctor.

Another option is to contact a reputable cancer clinic or teaching hospital for help in getting a second opinion. Look for National Cancer Institute (NCI)-designated comprehensive cancer centers, which are recognized by the federal government for quality care. The Mayo Clinic Comprehensive Cancer Center is one such center. You also can call the NCI's Cancer Information Service at 800-4-CANCER or visit livehelp.cancer.gov.

Keep in mind that the costs for obtaining a second opinion may vary. To save time and money in the long run, check with your insurance company to see what your plan covers before making an appointment. See Chapter 12 for more information about finances and insurance.

It's also important to seek a second opinion if you're having difficulty connecting with your primary oncology team. If you don't feel comfortable with the people on your team, you are entitled to search for others with whom you can build a more productive relationship.

Sometimes, finding a second opinion can feel too overwhelming to pursue. See if you can enlist a friend or family member to help you do some research online, make phone calls and go with you to medical appointments to take notes and ask questions. Simply having someone organize all your information — tumor details, treatment plans, medications, other conditions and so on — in one folder can be helpful in assessing your options.

You may not want to get a second opinion, and that's OK, too. If you have confidence in the judgment of your health care team or have researched your cancer and are comfortable with your treatment plan, you may decide to forgo a second opinion.

anger can destroy paths to happiness that you otherwise might find. In addition, anger can consume energy
and contribute to depression.

Exercising, talking with someone you trust or
sorting through your thoughts in writing may help
you work through feelings of anger and resentment. If
you need additional help, reach out to a therapist or
social worker, or ask your health care team for the
name of a mental health professional.

Sadness and depression
You may be mourning the life you knew and feeling
overwhelming sadness that you might not be able to
accomplish all that you had planned, or see your loved
ones reach significant milestones, such as college
graduations or retirement. Depression can leave you
feeling hopeless or numb. You may cry more than you
usually do, feel unmotivated or have the urge to pull
away from family and friends. Sleep can be disrupted,
and you may feel a lack of energy.

Given what you're going through, feeling sad is
entirely normal. You may find little ways to slowly work
through your emotions and care for yourself, such as
leaning on the support of friends and family, being in
nature, or enrolling in an art or exercise class that
makes you feel better. Sometimes, it helps to know
you're not alone. Nonprofit organizations such as Living
Beyond Breast Cancer or Young Survival Coalition
often share stories online or offer virtual meeting
places where you can learn about people living with
metastatic breast cancer and how they are coping
with the challenges they meet.

Sometimes, feelings of sadness and apathy run
deeper. In these cases, it's essential to talk to your
doctor or another member of your health care team.
Talking with a psychologist or counselor can be an

effective way to help you cope. In some cases, taking an antidepressant can be helpful.

Loneliness

Even though family and friends do their best to understand what you're going through, it's impossible to really "get it" unless they've been through it too. After your diagnosis of metastatic breast cancer, you may even notice that you see less of some people as they struggle to come to terms with your situation. Sometimes, people fear that they'll say the wrong thing or feel awkward around you.

If you miss the presence of family members or friends, reach out and let them know. You might want to take the lead in the conversation and share the things that you feel comfortable talking about. Some people may hold back, feeling they can't talk about what's going on in their lives because it sounds too minor compared to what you're going through. Let them know it's OK to talk about other things or that your sense of humor is still quite intact. Being vulnerable and honest together is good for your overall well-being and for your relationship.

Support groups, either in-person or virtual, can be beneficial too, as they provide the opportunity to connect with others who are in similar situations as yourself. Some cancer survivors consider support groups a positive aspect of a cancer diagnosis, as they meet people they might not have crossed paths with otherwise. For many people — though not all — their network of fellow breast cancer survivors is a place of comfort and support.

Forced positivity

It may be tempting to put on a happy face in front of others so that you don't worry your family and friends or seem too negative. But *pretending* to feel better doesn't always result in *actually* feeling better.

Some people with cancer may avoid addressing cancer concerns because they fear that perceived negativity will make them sicker. Well-meaning friends and family may also encourage them to be more positive. While staying hopeful is undoubtedly good, it's important to accept your feelings, whatever they may be, as they come — and to express yourself as needed.

While everyone copes differently, over time you may find that your feelings change.

You may find emotional and physical strength that you didn't know you had.

'MY CANCER IS BACK'

Often, another significant source of stress for people with metastatic breast cancer is determining how to tell loved ones and friends that the cancer has spread and is no longer curable. There's no right or wrong way to approach the conversation. Look for a time when you won't be interrupted and you'll have plenty of time to talk and discuss what comes next.

Talking about your diagnosis with family and friends

Breaking the news of your diagnosis to family and friends can cause intense emotional reactions from your loved ones. Because this is already a stressful time for you, consider choosing one person close to you to tell first and have that person be there to support you when you share the news with others. This person may also be the one you ask to provide medical updates to others or delegate tasks if you need help.

It may take a little while for others to fully understand — for example, some medical terms, such as metastatic, may need to be explained — but once your loved ones have had time to process the news, consider talking about ways they may be able to support you. This may be emotional support or help with daily needs, such as driving you to treatment, grocery shopping or picking up your kids from school.

Be prepared for different reactions. Most likely, people will be eager to help in whatever way you need. But there may be some who aren't able to help you as you'd assumed or hoped. This can be upsetting, but it's probably not about you. Maybe they're avoiding you because they have painful memories of a loved one who died of cancer or because they simply don't know how to deal with the news. In any case, you can focus instead on all the love and support you're getting from those people who *are* willing and able to help.

Talking about your diagnosis with a spouse or partner
Learning about a partner's diagnosis of metastatic breast cancer can have a deep impact on a person's life. Taking your time to discuss the diagnosis, finding out what to expect and outlining what your roles might look like as you move forward can be comforting to both of you. Chapter 13 has information specifically for spouses and partners of breast cancer survivors.

Going to medical appointments together can help your partner learn more about your experience and treatment and take some of the mystery — and fear — out of your diagnosis. Having frank discussions about what the future holds can help prepare your partner for what can be an overwhelming time. For example, your spouse or partner may need to take on most of the household chores while you adjust to treatment. If you need to quit your job, your spouse or partner may have to work extra hours or find a way to cut back on expenses.

WHAT YOU CAN DO

Metastatic breast cancer care can sometimes feel like it's all about what's being done to you, rather than what you can do for yourself. But there is something that you can do and that is to keep moving. Research shows that staying physically active when you have metastatic breast cancer is one of the most important ways you can increase the quality of your life. Regular physical activity can help improve your energy levels, mood, and how well you sleep.

There's no need to join an extreme fitness program. Do something that you enjoy. Walking for 30 minutes a day or keeping up with a favorite hobby such as gardening or playing tennis is enough to provide you with anti-cancer health benefits. If you have bone metastases, however, check in with your oncologist or primary care provider about safe activities that reduce your risk of fracture.

See Chapter 3 for more information on habits that can help you stay healthy and reduce cancer's effects on your life.

It's also natural for a partner to worry about intimacy and sex moving forward (see Chapter 9). Your partner may feel guilty for wanting to connect with you sexually when you're tired, or they may worry about hurting you. Open and honest discussions about how you're feeling, and finding alternative ways to be sexually intimate — such as with touch or cuddling — allow you to maintain a connection.

For some partners, fear stemming from a diagnosis or anxiety about taking on a caregiving role may manifest as anger, resentment or hyper-vigilance, which can add to an already stressful situation. If this is the case, consider suggesting that your spouse or partner meet with a therapist experienced in helping people who are coping with life-threatening illnesses. Going solo to therapy appointments may create space for your significant other to be open without fear of being insensitive or hurting your feelings.

It is essential to keep the lines of communication open and talk about possible solutions to issues as they arise.

Talking about your diagnosis with your children

For many people with metastatic cancer, talking to their children about the cancer can feel almost impossible. How do you begin? It may help to become more comfortable with your diagnosis first, or at least to have begun the process of absorbing it, before telling your children.

How you approach your children largely depends on their age. The important thing is to be as truthful as possible, using words you think they will understand. Even if they don't completely comprehend what you're saying, children often know something is going on, and that can be frightening at a young age, especially if it appears to be a secret. Here are some tips for addressing your diagnosis of metastatic breast cancer:

- Explain that while your cancer can't be cured, some treatments may be able to help you feel better and live longer.
- Reinforce with younger children that cancer isn't contagious, nor is it the result of something they did.

- Consider enlisting the help of a counselor or someone close to the family with whom teenagers can talk honestly and openly about what's going on, especially if they have been lashing out or exhibiting signs of anger or fear. Although older children can usually handle more specific information, this is still a wrenching situation and most likely they will find it very difficult to process.
- Prepare children for changes to everyday routines. For example, you may be too tired on some days to attend soccer practice, so another family member will take over. On other days, you may be too tired to make dinner, so someone else will make it or deliver it. Let them know what's coming, so there are no upsetting surprises.
- Reassure them that you'll keep them updated on any changes and that you're always available for follow-up questions.
- Suggest trusted websites you can look at together if they want more information. Remember that some of these sites may mention survival statistics, which can be confusing or upsetting. One way to explain statistics is to say that these numbers are based on large groups of people, and they don't necessarily reflect what will happen to you. Given the pace of new therapies being made available through research, today's statistics are likely to already be outdated.
- Watch for outward signs of anxiety in younger children, which may appear as physical symptoms such as headaches or stomachaches.
- It may be helpful to involve your younger child's school, outside care provider, or health care team to make sure your child receives the necessary support.
- Schedule time to have fun together, such as watching movies or playing board games.

Parenting is difficult enough when you don't have metastatic breast cancer. But managing a diagnosis of metastatic cancer while raising kids can be physically and emotionally exhausting in ways you never anticipated.

When faced with difficult circumstances, children's behavior can shift from their usual patterns to being more clingy, impulsive, distant or withdrawn. Express willingness to talk about your child's feelings and to assure them that no matter what happens, your love doesn't change and you're doing everything you can to be around for as long as possible.

It's not uncommon for people with cancer to worry that their diagnosis is upsetting or burdening their loved ones. However, most often, family and friends want to listen and want to help. These times can create beautiful bonds between you and those you love. And it can benefit those providing support, allowing them to find more meaning and purpose in their lives.

FINDING ACCEPTANCE

Most people with metastatic breast cancer eventually reach a point of acceptance. This may not mean that you're OK with your diagnosis or that the anger or sadness you experienced because of the cancer is gone. You'll still have bad days. Instead, it means you've arrived at a place where you understand your circumstances, and you're adjusting your life to this new reality. During this time, you'll probably find it easier to make decisions about your future, such as creating advance directives or legacy items. (See "Leaving a legacy" on page 205.)

Many people diagnosed with advanced cancer start digging deeper into their values, looking for purpose and thinking about what kind of legacy they want to leave. You may look back on what's happened in your life. You may want to make peace with something or someone from your past. Sometimes people turn to religion or faith. Others may volunteer or become advocates for the metastatic breast cancer community.

It's not uncommon for values to change and for you to begin realizing what matters most. Suddenly, for example, cleaning the house seems much less important than a day trip with the family. You may take more time off from work and experience some of the items on your bucket list. Metastatic breast cancer may provide greater clarity about what's important and what's not worth losing sleep over.

With acceptance often comes hope. Where cancer made you feel you had no control over your life, learning to accept your situation and make decisions about your future can be empowering.

6

Maximizing quality of life with palliative care

Palliative care is a specialty that focuses on managing symptoms of cancer and any side effects caused by treatment. The goal of palliative care is to improve quality of life. Palliative care aims to address not only physical symptoms, such as pain, but also the emotional, social and spiritual effects of cancer on your life. It also supports the needs of your family members and caregivers.

PALLIATIVE CARE IS NOT HOSPICE CARE

Palliative care is not the same as hospice care. Palliative care is appropriate for people with any stage of cancer. Ideally, it should be introduced as close to the time of your diagnosis as possible. Effectively managing your symptoms not only improves your quality of life but also may improve your ability to receive your medical treatments on time and at full dose. The American Society of Clinical Oncology recommends early palliative care for all people with advanced cancer.

Hospice care is solely focused on people who have a more limited prognosis. It is appropriate when goals of care move from treatment of cancer to focus on treatment of symptoms and optimizing quality of life (see page 207).

Examples of palliative care include pain management, nutritional support, counseling, exercise, music therapy and meditation. Other symptoms such as nausea, constipation, cough and fatigue can also be effectively managed with palliative care.

Palliative care is a team-based approach to care. Your team may include the primary palliative care doctor, nurses, social workers and chaplains. The goal is for the team to work together in managing your symptoms, but also in providing more specific support of your emotional, social and spiritual needs. Your palliative care team can also help you prepare an advance

WILL MY INSURANCE COVER PALLIATIVE CARE?

Private insurers, Medicare and Medicaid usually pay for supportive and palliative care services. Medicaid coverage varies by state. If you're unsure about your coverage, reach out to your insurance company or a social worker or financial counselor where you receive treatment.

WHAT IS INTEGRATIVE ONCOLOGY?

Integrative oncology is an area of cancer care that aims to help people cope with the stress of a cancer diagnosis and address symptoms caused by the disease and its treatment, such as fatigue, pain, nausea, anxiety and other effects. The practice combines conventional Western medicine with evidence-based complementary treatments. That means the treatments have been researched and proved to be safe and effective in healing.

Integrative oncologists counsel people receiving cancer treatment on practices that can help relieve side effects and improve treatment outcomes. They help cancer patients adopt a healthy lifestyle and lose weight, understand which herbal and dietary supplements are safe to take, and recommend integrative medicine practices that might help manage a person's symptoms.

Examples of evidence-based techniques are acupuncture and acupressure, aromatherapy, meditation, music therapy, exercise and movement, massage, Reiki, yoga, tai chi, retraining sleep habits, and stress and anxiety management.

Integrative medicine is now being used at many cancer centers. If your cancer care team doesn't have an integrative oncologist on staff, ask if there's an integrative medicine program in your area that can help.

directive and create a care plan that aligns with your treatment goals and personal values.

Those who pursue palliative care often experience an improvement in symptoms, including a decrease in depression and anxiety. In addition, they have a better overall quality of life and usually are more satisfied with their treatment. In some cases, palliative care can even extend survival.

Palliative care for cancer is offered at most major hospitals or cancer clinics. If you haven't been offered palliative care, talk to your oncologist. If it's not available where you receive cancer care, there may be other ways to get some of the same benefits. For example, oncology nurses often have a lot of experience helping people with cancer feel better and may be able to offer specific recommendations for problems you're facing. Your primary care doctor may be able to help you with symptom relief and provide a referral to a mental health counselor. In addition, you may be able to connect with helpful resources online. For a list of additional resources, see page 209.

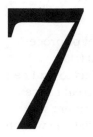

7

Clinical trials

Clinical trials are an important part of breast cancer treatment at all phases of care. A clinical trial can be a game changer if you find one that's a good fit for you. A clinical trial is not a last resort. Joining a clinical trial can give you access to experimental treatment options that may be effective but are not yet approved by the Food and Drug Administration (FDA). In addition, there are clinical trials that examine quality-of-life issues after treatment.

Importantly, your participation helps researchers improve cancer care for future patients. This is a promising time in breast cancer research, with many new treatments under study and continuous refinements to existing treatments.

WHAT IS A CLINICAL TRIAL?

Research studies that evaluate a treatment or procedure and involve people are called clinical trials.

Cancer researchers design clinical trials to find new and better ways to diagnose, control and treat cancer, and to manage cancer symptoms and treatment side effects. When participating in a clinical trial you will be guaranteed to receive standard treatment if you do not receive the treatment being evaluated. When clinical trials demonstrate better results than standard treatment, the trial treatment becomes the standard.

People who volunteer to participate in clinical trials help researchers test new medicines, procedures, techniques and devices. Researchers also use clinical trials to test new ways of using existing treatments, as well as lifestyle and behavior changes.

Joining a clinical trial can give you earlier access to new treatments in all phases of development. Participating in a trial doesn't mean your health care team has given up on your getting well. And it doesn't make you an experiment or number. Treatment for cancer has improved significantly in the past few decades, and many of today's advances were discovered through yesterday's clinical trials.

PHASES OF INVESTIGATION

For a new cancer treatment to become standard, it usually goes through two or three phases of a clinical trial. The early phases of cancer clinical trials are designed to study the safety of the new treatment. Later phases determine the effectiveness of the new treatment while continuing to study its safety.

Phase I

The goals of a phase I clinical trial, also called an early-phase clinical trial, are to determine safe dosage levels and safe methods of delivering a new treatment. An early-phase clinical trial might be the first time an experimental cancer drug or intervention is used with people.

Phase II

The goals of a phase II cancer clinical trial are to evaluate the effectiveness of the cancer treatment and to monitor side effects. While side effects are monitored in all phases of clinical trials, they are a special focus in phase II.

Phase III

The goal of a phase III cancer clinical trial is to compare the new treatment to the standard treatment.

Phase IV

The goal of a phase IV cancer clinical trial is to further assess the long-term safety and effectiveness of a treatment. A phase IV clinical trial is conducted after FDA approval.

WHO SHOULD PARTICIPATE IN A CANCER CLINICAL TRIAL?

Clinical trials are generally available for all stages of breast cancer. They are an important option to think about any time you or someone you love needs cancer treatment.

It's particularly important to think about a clinical trial if you are part of a racial or ethnic minority patient group. Too often, participants in clinical studies tend to be overwhelmingly — or disproportionately — white. Diversity in clinical trials is critical for responsible science and better medicine. When more people from more diverse groups participate in clinical trials, researchers can be more confident that promising new treatments work for everyone.

Researchers at Mayo Clinic and elsewhere are committed to addressing barriers that keep historically marginalized groups from enrolling in clinical trials. Lack of trust is one barrier, based on past acts of medical racism and abuse, such as the Tuskegee Study and the story of Henrietta Lacks. Even today, bias and incorrect assumptions play a role, as members of minority groups aren't always invited to join a research study, even when appropriate. In a recent study, nearly half of Black women with metastatic cancer reported that they never received information about participation in a clinical trial.

While the medical field works to address these health care disparities, you can still advocate for yourself by insisting on information about clinical trials that are available to you — and considering them seriously.

HOW CAN YOU FIND A CLINICAL TRIAL?

Talk to your oncologist. Your oncologist may be involved in a clinical trial that is right for you or may refer you to another principal investigator.

You can also find clinical trials at these resources:

- www.cancer.gov
- www.clinicaltrials.gov
- www.mayo.edu/research/clinical-trials

WHAT QUESTIONS SHOULD YOU ASK BEFORE AGREEING TO PARTICIPATE?

You should be well-informed and comfortable before making any decisions about taking part in a clinical trial. Here are some questions to discuss with your care team and the clinical trial team:

- What is the goal of the trial?
- Why might this study be right for me?
- What tests or treatments are involved?
- What are the benefits, risks or inconveniences?
- Does my participation prevent me from receiving other types of treatment now or in the future?
- Will I have to pay for travel or lodging expenses or other costs?
- How much travel is necessary? Can I participate through my local provider or telehealth services?
- How long will the study last?

In some cases, you may be able to connect with former or current trial participants who volunteer to talk with people considering a study. If travel or cost are obstacles to your participation, ask to speak to the clinical trial coordinator or a patient navigator. They may have access to financial and other resources to assist you.

Remember: If you explore clinical trial options, you don't have to sign up, even if you qualify. And, if you choose to join a clinical trial, you can opt out at any time, for any reason.

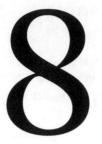

Integrative therapies

Interest in therapies outside the range of conventional medical treatments has increased substantially in recent years — not just among the public but in the medical community as well. People not only want to treat cancer, but they also want a good quality of life.

For a while, unconventional therapies were referred to as alternative medicine. That's because these types of treatments were seen as alternatives to conventional medicine — and many medical professionals, worried that these alternatives might interfere with or be used instead of proven cancer treatments, warned against them.

But as evidence of safety and effectiveness grows, many such therapies are now being integrated with conventional medicine in an effort to treat the whole person — body, mind and spirit. Thus, the term *alternative* has been dropped, and these therapies are now called complementary and integrative medicine or simply integrative medicine.

Integrative medicine combines the most well-researched, evidence-based conventional medicine with the most well-researched, evidence-based complementary therapies to achieve the appropriate care for each person.

This chapter focuses primarily on therapies that might aid your recovery from cancer treatment. The therapies mentioned here are known to be generally safe. They may help improve the quality of your life by relieving pain, boosting your energy, and reducing stress or anxiety. If you're looking for information about dietary supplements, turn to page 43.

MINDFULNESS

Your state of mind can and does influence your physical body. For example, when you are upset or anxious, your blood pressure may increase or you may start to feel lightheaded. Stress can affect your emotions, your behaviors, your enjoyment of life, and even some of your physiologic responses, such as heart rate or breathing.

Learning how to calm the mind can be beneficial to your health and well-being. This is why mindfulness-based techniques are typically at the top the list of integrative therapies that doctors think are helpful for breast cancer survivors.

But what exactly is mindfulness? At its simplest, mindfulness involves staying focused on the present moment. It requires you to focus your awareness on what you're experiencing in an open, curious and nonjudgmental way.

The goal of mindfulness is to create distance between how you view or experience certain situations or feelings and how you respond to them. For example, instead of getting caught up in worries about an upcoming medical appointment, you might step back and simply observe the thoughts and emotions that are coming up for you. This moment of nonjudgmental awareness gives you the space to move forward more thoughtfully and calmly.

Mindfulness-based therapies
Many cancer survivors benefit from attending a structured, evidence-based program in which trained experts teach formal and informal mindfulness techniques. Examples of these techniques may include body scan meditation, gentle yoga, sitting and walking meditation, and breathing exercises.

One well-established program is called mindfulness-based stress reduction (MBSR). MBSR is an evidence-based course that typically takes place over 6 to 8 weeks. Participants engage in weekly group sessions lasting 2 to 3 hours. A one-day retreat near the end of the program may also be included. In recent years, MBSR has been adapted for cancer survivors, including mindfulness-based cancer recovery (MBCR) and mindfulness-based stress reduction for breast cancer, or MBSR(BC).

These mindfulness-based programs can take place in person or online. Health care clinics, universities, community-based meditations centers, and other local or online organizations may offer this therapy. You can ask your health care team for a recommendation.

Research on cancer survivors who have gone through MBSR and other mindfulness-based programs shows that these structured interventions may help to:
• Decrease stress.
• Reduce fatigue.

- Lessen depression and anxiety.
- Improve sleep.
- Reduce pain due to treatment-related neuropathy.

In some cancer survivors, mindfulness-based interventions may lead to greater personal growth in the aftermath of a cancer diagnosis and treatment. This phenomenon is sometimes called post-traumatic growth (see page 26). It involves finding positive meaning in a traumatic experience. Cancer survivors who experience post-traumatic growth might enjoy greater confidence and inner strength, an increased appreciation for life, closer relationships or a greater connection to their spirituality.

Mindfulness exercises
If enrolling in a structured mindfulness-based program isn't feasible, you can practice focused exercises on your own.

Set aside some time each day when you can be in a quiet place without distractions or interruptions. You might choose to practice this type of exercise early in the morning before you begin your daily routine or at night before going to bed. Try practicing mindfulness every day for about six months. Over time, you might find that it becomes more effortless and natural.

Body scan meditation
Lie on your back with your legs extended and arms at your sides, palms facing up. Focus your attention slowly and deliberately on each part of your body, in order, from toe to head or head to toe. Be aware of any sensations, emotions or thoughts associated with each part of your body.

Sitting meditation

Sit comfortably in a chair with your back straight, feet flat on the floor and hands in your lap. Breathing through your nose, focus on your breath moving in and out of your body. If physical sensations or thoughts interrupt your meditation, note the experience and then return your focus to your breath. If you're new to meditation, many digital apps provide guided meditations that you can follow.

Walking meditation

Find a quiet indoor or outdoor space 10 to 20 feet in length and begin to walk slowly. Focus on the experience of walking, being aware of the sensations of standing and the subtle movements that keep your balance. When you reach the end of your path, turn and continue walking, maintaining awareness of your sensations.

Yoga

Yoga involves moving through a series of body postures while practicing controlled breathing exercises. A gentle form of yoga known as Hatha yoga may be particularly beneficial for breast cancer survivors. Along with providing the benefits of mindful movement, Hatha yoga may improve flexibility and range of motion after breast cancer surgery.

You can do yoga alone or in a group, and it doesn't require a big investment to get started. You might begin by taking a class or following yoga videos online. Then, after you become adept at the postures and breathing, continue the practice at home on your own.

Tai chi

Tai chi is a graceful form of exercise that involves a series of movements performed in a slow, focused

> Over the years, I continued my practice of tai chi and my schedule of art. The deep breathing and slow movement of tai chi was healing, as was the joy I felt doing art with the community of my class. The COVID years interfered with some of these classes, but I continued on my own. — P. W.

---

manner and accompanied by deep breathing. Often described as meditation in motion, tai chi promotes serenity through gentle, flowing movements. Although you can use videos and books to learn how to do tai chi, consider seeking guidance from a qualified tai chi instructor to gain the activity's full benefits and learn proper techniques. Check for tai chi classes at your local community center, gym or martial arts school.

Qigong
Closely related to tai chi, qigong combines mindful breathing, meditation and slow, rhythmic movements. Qigong is commonly performed standing, but some forms are done in sitting or lying-down positions. If possible, you may want to start out with the guidance of an experienced instructor.

ACUPUNCTURE

Acupuncture is one of the most researched and accepted forms of integrative medicine. It involves inserting hair-thin needles into the skin at strategic points in the body. A key component of traditional Chinese medicine,

SPIRITUALITY AND CANCER

While the spiritual side of humans — the part that understands love and seeks to find meaning and purpose in life — is universally recognized, it hasn't always been addressed in discussions of health, particularly in modern Western medicine. This might be because of historical efforts to separate medicine from practices with little evidence of health benefits. But the medical field increasingly acknowledges that spiritual elements do play an important part in the overall health of many people. For some people with metastatic cancer, their faith in God or a higher power is a source of great comfort and strength, especially in times of distress or even doubt.

The word spirituality is often used interchangeably with religion, but the terms are not the same. Spirituality can mean vastly different things to people with different beliefs and faith traditions. For some, spirituality flows from religious experiences. For others, spirituality is connected to nature and feeling in tune with oneself and the universe. Still, for others, spirituality is expressed through relationships, service, music, meditation or art. Many people find meaning and purpose through a combination of these things.

A cancer diagnosis may change your views on spirituality. You may find that your spiritual intel-

acupuncture may provide relief for common side effects and symptoms experienced after cancer treatment.

Many studies have examined the use of acupuncture on cancer survivors. The benefits of this ligence becomes stronger and deeper from the challenges you have overcome. Or you may feel abandoned and struggling to maintain faith because of your circumstances. It's common to experience a wide range of both negative and positive feelings.

Science is finding that nurturing your spiritual well-being can positively influence the quality of your life and your ability to cope with your illness. You can cultivate your spirituality by:

- Attending religious services or participating in a faith community.
- Engaging in prayer, meditation, mindfulness or relaxation practices to help focus your thoughts and find peace of mind.
- Keeping a journal to help you express your feelings and record your thoughts.
- Talking to others whose spiritual lives you admire; asking questions to learn how they found their way to a fulfilling spiritual life.
- Making a difference by volunteering in your community.
- Talking with your spiritual or religious leader to help guide you through some of the questions raised by your illness.

therapy are sometimes difficult to measure, but evidence suggests acupuncture may reduce a range of cancer-related symptoms, including:

> **My biggest strength during my breast cancer journey has been my faith and the ability to maintain a sense of HOPE that no matter what happens, I'll be okay. I also believe that a little dose of humor goes a long way in relieving anxiety, stress and tension. — L. K.**

- Pain.
- Fatigue.
- Hot flashes.
- Nerve problems, also called neuropathy.
- Depression.
- Anxiety.
- Sleep problems.

How it works
Traditional Chinese medicine explains acupuncture as a technique for balancing the flow of energy or life force — known as chi or qi (chee) — that is believed to flow through pathways (meridians) in your body. By inserting needles at specific points along these meridians, acupuncture practitioners believe that your energy flow will re-balance.

In contrast, many Western practitioners view the acupuncture points as places to stimulate nerves, muscles and connective tissue. Some believe that this stimulation boosts your body's natural painkillers.

What to expect
During an acupuncture session, an acupuncturist inserts between five and 20 sterile needles into specific points on your body while you sit or lie on a padded table. Most people feel only minimal pain or pressure as the needles are inserted; some feel nothing at all.

Once the needles are in place, you generally shouldn't feel any pain. Significant pain is a sign that the procedure isn't being performed properly. Your acupuncturist may gently move or twirl the needles after placement or apply heat or mild electrical pulses to the needles. There is usually no discomfort when the needles are removed.

The number of acupuncture sessions needed differs from person to person and depends on how severe your symptoms are. It's common to receive 6 to 8 treatments, and these often occur once per week. You should experience some relief within the first few weeks. If your symptoms don't start to improve, consider discussing other treatment options with your primary care doctor.

Risks and side effects

The risks of acupuncture are low if you're working with a competent, certified acupuncturist. Common side effects include soreness or minor bleeding or bruising where the needles were inserted. Single-use, disposable needles are now the practice standard, so the risk of infection is small.

It's important to work with someone who has been trained and certified. Check the acupuncturist's training and credentials. Most states require that acupuncturists who aren't physicians pass an exam conducted by the National Certification Commission for Acupuncture and Oriental Medicine.

MASSAGE

From birth, the warm touch of other human beings provides comfort and pleasure. So it seems reasonable to assume that massage and other therapies like it can contribute to improved quality of life for breast cancer survivors.

Benefits of massage therapy include relaxation and decreased muscle tension. Studies on cancer survivors indicate that massage therapy may help improve symptoms such as:

- Anxiety.
- Pain.
- Stress.
- Fatigue.
- Sleep problems.

Types of massage therapy used in cancer care include Swedish massage, foot or hand massage (reflexology), application of light pressure at specific points on the body (acupressure), and focused pressure and stretching (myofascial release therapy). One type of massage-like technique called manual lymph drainage uses precise light rhythmic motions to reduce swelling of the arm after a mastectomy.

Talk with your health care team about whether massage is safe for you and what areas of your body, if any, the massage therapist should avoid. Be sure your massage therapist graduated from an accredited program and meets state licensing requirements. If possible, look for a massage therapist who's received additional training in massage techniques for people with cancer. Ask your oncologist for a recommendation. Or check the Society for Oncology Massage, which lists recommended practitioners on its website.

Massage has very few risks if done by a qualified professional. If you have a massage, make sure the massage therapist knows which parts of your body were radiated or underwent surgery so that they can use care in those areas. If it's not applied carefully, vigorous massage may cause further harm to tissue that has already been damaged by surgery or radiation therapy.

HYPNOSIS

Hypnosis is a changed state of awareness and increased relaxation. Also called hypnotherapy, hypnosis usually is done with the guidance of a hypnosis specialist using verbal repetition and mental images.

Hypnosis may help relieve symptoms such as:

- Pain.
- Hot flashes.
- Fatigue.
- Anxiety.

What to expect

A hypnosis specialist typically begins the process by talking in a gentle, soothing tone, describing images that create a sense of relaxation, security and well-being. When you're relaxed and calm, the specialist suggests ways for you to achieve your goals. That may include, for example, ways to ease pain or reduce hot flashes. The provider also may help you visualize vivid, meaningful mental images of yourself accomplishing your goals.

When the session is over, you may be able to bring yourself out of hypnosis on your own, or the hypnosis specialist may help you gradually and comfortably increase your alertness.

Over time, you may be able to practice self-hypnosis. During self-hypnosis, you reach a state of relaxation and calm without another person's guidance. This skill can be helpful in many situations, such as before medical appointments or procedures.

> I adopted a dog shortly after surgery. It forced me to get out of bed on days I did not want to. Not an official therapy dog, but my therapy dog. — L. M.

Hypnosis done by a trained specialist is a safe treatment. Keep in mind, though, that hypnosis isn't right for everyone. Not all people are able to enter a state of hypnosis fully enough for it to work well. In general, the more quickly and easily you can reach a state of relaxation and calm during a session, the more likely it is that you'll benefit from hypnosis.

Be sure to choose a health care specialist who is certified to perform hypnosis. Get a recommendation from your primary care doctor or someone on your cancer care team. Or ask for a recommendation from someone you trust.

MEDICAL CANNABIS

Medical cannabis refers to herbal products derived from the Cannabis sativa plant that are used to ease symptoms caused by medical conditions. Cannabis sativa contains many active compounds called cannabinoids. The best-known cannabinoids are delta-9-tetrahydrocannabinol (THC) and cannabidiol (CBD). THC is the primary ingredient in marijuana that makes people "high." CBD doesn't have this effect.

In the United States, most states allow CBD- and THC-based products to be used for medical reasons. In contrast, federal law prohibits the use of whole plant Cannabis sativa or its derivatives for any purpose.

However, CBD derived from the hemp plant (less than 0.3% THC) is legal under federal law.

Uses
Ongoing research into medical cannabis indicates that it may help reduce these common symptoms:

- **Pain** One of the most common medical uses of cannabis is to reduce pain, including chronic nerve (neuropathic) pain. Research suggests that products containing a combination of THC and CBD may be more effective for short-term pain relief than CBD alone.
- **Sleep problems** Medical cannabis may slightly improve sleep quality, particularly if sleep problems are caused by chronic pain. Low-dose CBD products for sleep problems are generally safe and may help if anxiety is contributing to poor sleep. However, for pain or nausea that contributes to poor sleep, adding in THC is generally needed. There are risks associated with adding in THC, which should be discussed with a knowledgeable provider.
- **Mental health** Some people report that CBD reduces anxiety and helps with well-being. Scientists have researched the effects of CBD on anxiety and depression in animals but the research on effectiveness and safety in humans is limited.

Side effects and risks
Further research is needed to determine whether the long-term use of cannabis is safe, but there are known side effects. Cannabis can also interact with other medications you're taking, such as blood thinners. If you plan to use products containing cannabinoids, talk to your primary care doctor first.

CBD is often well-tolerated, but at higher doses it can cause side effects such as:

- Diarrhea.
- Reduced appetite.
- Drowsiness and fatigue.
- Potential for drug interactions.

Products containing THC may have more side effects, including:
- Increased heart rate.
- Dizziness.
- Impaired concentration and memory.
- Slower reaction times.
- Drug-to-drug interactions.
- Increased risk of heart attack and stroke.
- Increased appetite.
- Potential for addiction.
- Hallucinations or mental illness.
- Withdrawal symptoms.

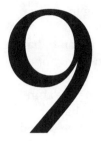

Sexual intimacy

During your cancer treatment, sex may have been a source of comfort, closeness and pleasure . . . or it may have been the last thing on your mind. Either way, you probably weren't focused on how treatment might affect your sex life further down the road.

Now that you're putting the puzzle pieces of your life back together, you may be wondering where sex fits in. How do you rekindle the romance or get back in the dating scene? Are the problems you're experiencing in the bedroom normal?

If you're asking these kinds of questions, you're in good company. Many cancer survivors are surprised to experience difficulties related to sex and intimacy after treatment. The issue of sex often gets overlooked by cancer care specialists, so it's understandable if you sometimes feel like you're stumbling along in silence and in the dark.

The first thing to know is that it's common to have concerns about your sex life after treatment. By one estimate, up to 75% of breast cancer survivors report sexual concerns. But just because problems are common doesn't mean they're inevitable. This chapter explains why you might be encountering some sexual health challenges and what you can do about it. With a positive approach and an open mind, you can find joy in your sex life.

HOW TREATMENT MAY AFFECT YOUR SEXUAL HEALTH

Surgery, chemotherapy, radiation and endocrine therapy — all of these can affect how you experience sex. Your emotions during recovery can play a role, too. Stress, worry, guilt or depression can put a damper on your sexual functioning — including libido, arousal and orgasms.

The way your cancer journey affects sexual intimacy may vary depending on your sex, gender, and sexual partners or relationship status. Here are some issues breast cancer survivors may experience:

Changes in the vaginal walls
Certain breast cancer treatments, including chemotherapy and endocrine therapy, can lead to a loss of estrogen. Lower estrogen levels can cause the tissues of the vulva and the vaginal walls to become less elastic, thinner, and more susceptible to bleeding, tearing and narrowing. Known as vulvovaginal atrophy, these changes can make sexual activity painful for many people.

Erectile dysfunction
A rare side effect of breast cancer treatment is the
inability to get or keep an erection firm enough for
sexual activity. This condition, called erectile dysfunction, is more common after radiation therapy or surgical interventions for prostate, bladder, colon or rectal
cancer. However, some people treated with chemotherapy or endocrine therapy may also develop this
condition.

Decreased sexual desire
If you experience treatment-related problems such as
vaginal pain due to vulvovaginal atrophy or erectile
dysfunction, your desire for sex may have declined. In
addition, chemotherapy and endocrine therapy can
disrupt your hormones, reducing libido. Your interest
in sex can also be diminished by emotions such as fear,
anxiety and sadness.

Another common culprit is appearance anxiety,
meaning worry related to body image. You may worry
about how your appearance has changed and may no
longer feel attractive or confident. People who have a
mastectomy are particularly vulnerable to this concern.
Removing an entire breast (mastectomy) or changing its
look and feel (lumpectomy) can affect your image of
yourself as a sexual being.

Difficulty with foreplay and reaching orgasm
If you were able to reach orgasm before cancer treatment, chances are pretty good you'll continue to do so
in the future. But the types of touch or stimulation that
used to excite you may no longer have the same effect.
For instance, foreplay in the past might have included
stroking your breasts or your nipples. If you've undergone a mastectomy, your breast area or nipples may
have lost some or all sensation. Being touched there

might also evoke complicated emotions that dampen arousal.

Keep in mind that your level of sensitivity in the nipple and breast area may continue to change as you recover from surgery. It may take up to a year to know what level of sensation you'll experience long-term.

Vulvovaginal atrophy can also impact your ability to reach orgasm. If the genital tissues aren't healthy, sensation and orgasmic function are often compromised. Pain during sex due to atrophy also reduces the likelihood of having an orgasm.

RESTORING YOUR SEXUAL WELLNESS

If you're experiencing post-treatment troubles with sexual intimacy, you might be uncomfortable talking about it. That's OK. This is often a difficult topic and not everyone feels comfortable discussing sexual concerns. It can be tempting to avoid any potential embarrassment by not talking about them. But voicing your concerns — even your nervousness about saying them out loud — is a crucial first step to regaining your sexual health. It might take some courage, but by confiding in your partner or seeking guidance from a health care professional, you may well be able to enjoy a satisfying sex life again. Talking things over with someone you trust can open the door to some creative solutions. Here are other steps you can take to restore your sexual health.

Eliminate vaginal pain during sex
If sex is painful due to dryness or other changes to vaginal tissues, don't try to just push through the pain. Pushing through sexual pain can cause damage and

often worsens both pain symptoms and sexual health outcomes in the long term. Instead, try these techniques:

Use a water-based lubricant
Lubricants can help reduce discomfort during sexual activity. They come in water-based or silicone-based formulas, or hybrids that contain both. Water-based lubricants often require repeat application during sexual activity but wash off easily with soap and water. Silicone lubricants last longer and may be used sparingly but don't wash off easily. If possible, look for organic products without glycerin or parabens, ingredients that can irritate the area outside the vagina (vulva).

Water-based lubricants are usually sold at drug stores and supermarkets. Silicone-based products and a greater variety of water-based lubricants are more typically available from websites, some medical suppliers and adult specialty stores. Experiment to find a product that you like. Just be sure to avoid petroleum jelly and other oil-based lubricants. They may make you more prone to yeast infections.

Extend nonpenetrative sexual activity
Make sure you're fully aroused before any attempts at penetrative sex. Extended touching and other types of nonpenetrative sexual stimulation allow your body to become more fully aroused and often serve to increase sexual desire.

Experiment with positions
Choose positions that allow for good mobility and, as needed, control of the pace and depth of penetrative sex. There are many ways to engage sexually. Be creative; explore ways that make you feel good.

TIPS FOR USING LUBRICANTS

Lubricants can help reduce discomfort during sex. Here are suggestions for using them:

- Place the lubricant in your vagina and the area outside and all around it before sex. Also apply it to anything that will penetrate the vagina, such as a penis, finger, dilator or vibrator.
- Glycerin is a common ingredient in water-based lubricants. If you have itching after their use, choose a silicone-based lubricant or a water-based lubricant that doesn't contain glycerin.
- Silicone-based lubricants are very slippery. If this product gets on the floor it may lead to falls.
- If your partner has erectile dysfunction, consider an alternative to silicone lubricants. The use of silicone lubricants may contribute to less friction and stimulation and may delay or reduce orgasm.
- Avoid silicone-based lubricants with vibrators or other sexual aids made of silicone. This type of lubricant may ruin vibrators, sexual aids or toys that contain silicone.

Practice deep breathing
Learning to breathe in a way that helps relax your muscles may help relieve discomfort or pain during sexual activities. Relaxed breathing also can help to improve your overall physical and mental health.

Speak up
If you experience pain or difficulty during sex, tell your partner. Take a break and allow yourself to relax. If the pain persists, brainstorm options for sexual pleasure that aren't painful.

Talk to your health care team
If sexual or genital pain continues to be a problem, pelvic floor physical therapy may help. A specialist in pelvic floor physical therapy can guide you in pelvic floor muscle relaxation techniques, stretching, deep breathing, and other approaches to reduce pain and improve sexual enjoyment.

For vaginal pain, vaginal dilators may be prescribed. These gently stretch your vaginal tissues and pelvic floor muscles. Vaginal dilators are lubricated latex, plastic or rubber cylinders that are made in a variety of sizes.

Seek help for erectile dysfunction
If you're experiencing erectile dysfunction, talk to someone on your health care team — even if you're embarrassed. This is not something you have to live with in silence. Medications or other direct treatments may help to resolve the issue. You can also explore new types of touch and stimulation to help you reach climax.

❝❝ Seek support from additional providers if you don't receive help from the first provider you speak with about your sexual health. Primary care providers and gynecologists aren't always as experienced in addressing sexual health after breast cancer treatment as specialized breast care providers. — L. H.

BOOST YOUR BODY IMAGE

Many breast cancer survivors experience negative feelings toward their bodies after treatment. How you feel about your body can affect your mood and overall well-being. It can also have a direct impact on your interest in sexual intimacy. Sex is less appealing if you don't feel sexy.

The good news is that breast cancer survivors report gaining greater body acceptance over time. But you don't have to wait for the future to arrive. Regardless of your gender or sexual orientation, you can take charge of your body image — and your sex life — now. Here are some suggestions that other breast cancer survivors have found helpful.

Get moving
Physical activity can help promote good self-esteem and a positive body image. Using your body for purposeful physical activity — be it participating in an aerobics class or walking on a trail — can shift your focus from how your body looks to what it can do.

Strut your stuff
Try a new haircut or hair color. Wear clothing, pajamas or lingerie that accentuates the parts of your body you do feel good about. One cancer survivor says she chooses "power outfits" when she's having a hard day. "I'll just put those on because it helps me feel more confident. Helps me rock it."

Seek out acceptance
How others view and treat you has a big effect on how you view yourself. Seek out people in your life who accept you for who you are. If possible, limit the time you spend with people who are overly focused on appearance.

Talk to other breast cancer survivors
Some people find it healing to share thoughts and feelings about their body image with other breast cancer survivors. It can be inspiring to hear from others who have learned ways to accept and appreciate their bodies.

Lean on your partner
If you're in a trusting relationship, let your partner know that you could use some encouragement. Partners in a healthy relationship want to be of help and will most likely appreciate the hint. Research on women breast cancer survivors reveals that when partners express positive feelings about their loved one's appearance, it can have a powerful effect on how they feel about themselves.

Be kind to yourself
Instead of dwelling on how cancer has changed your appearance, try refocusing your lens on your strengths. As one breast cancer survivor put it, "I consider that I've been through a lot and my body has been through a lot. So I give praise to myself." This type of gratitude and self-compassion can extend beyond your body. Think about what's going well in your life and what you're thankful for.

Rediscover your body
If you're having difficulties feeling aroused or reaching orgasm, one technique to try is body mapping. Also called pleasure mapping, it involves relearning your body sensations and erogenous zones through exploratory touch. Some people prefer to engage in body mapping on their own before sharing what they've learned with a partner. Other people enjoy body mapping with a partner.

You might also try experimenting with different types of stimulation, such as vibration, pressure, or suction. For example, try using a hand-held vibrator on your genitals or other erogenous areas. Some breast cancer survivors who have lost sensation in the breast area or nipples find that they're able to experience pleasurable sensations by using a strong suction-style vibrator on that part of the body. Researchers are working on new treatments to restore lost sensation after breast cancer surgery.

RECONNECT WITH YOUR PARTNER

If you're in a relationship, one of the best ways to improve sexual intimacy is to open the lines of communication. After breast cancer treatment, many couples get caught in a harmful cycle of silence around sex. Each person assumes they know what the other is thinking: *She doesn't feel close to me anymore. He dislikes my body. They no longer find me attractive.* These unspoken assumptions can lead to misunderstandings, hurt feelings and a growing chasm between you and your partner.

Have a conversation

Talking out loud about the issue, awkward as it may feel, can help clear the air and renew emotional and physical intimacy. If you're wanting to reconnect sexually, begin by letting your partner know. Revealing those feelings can help break down some of the barriers that might have arisen between you. Keep the conversation going by sharing some thoughts and desires you have about your sex life. Ask about what hopes and wishes your partner may have. Try to stay open and positive — you've been through a lot.

Be patient
You may feel shy about reconnecting sexually, especially if you haven't had sex for a while. Remember that it's not a race. Give yourselves permission to take things as slowly as you need to, communicating as you go. And don't forget to have fun along the way — or even a few laughs. It's easy to get too serious about sex. A good chuckle about a sexy move gone awry can break the ice and bring you closer.

Set aside time for romance
When you're ready, make a date with your partner. Create a sensual mood using lighting, music, fragrance or all of the above. Take your time, focusing on pleasure and arousal. Slowly reacquaint yourself with your partner. Agreeing not to include certain sexual activities, such as intercourse, right away, can help you relax and slowly ease back into sexual intimacy with less anxiety.

Be open to experimentation
You and your partner may need to take time to explore what feels good to you and what doesn't — without an end goal of reaching orgasm. You can also try experimenting with different sexual positions or using sexual aids, such as a vibrator.

Sexual fantasy may be another way to rediscover pleasure in the bedroom. Before or during sexual intimacy, try playing out a fantasy in your head or with your partner. This can help get you in the mood and refocus your mind away from negative thoughts.

Redefine sexual pleasure
Many people equate sex to penetration during intercourse. If that type of sexual activity has become uncomfortable, you or your partner may feel

disappointed or frustrated. If sex is painful, it's important to stop what you're doing. But that doesn't mean you have to stop being sexual together. Instead of giving up, explore nonpainful ways to give and receive pleasure. Enjoy sexual pleasure through kissing, stroking, hugging and cuddling.

Consider working with a sex therapist
Sometimes, behavioral and psychological support from a qualified sex therapist is helpful for navigating sexual health challenges after cancer. Therapy may focus on improving communication skills, addressing body image concerns, or practicing techniques to decrease anxiety and increase satisfaction during sex. A sex therapist may provide education about improving the sexual experience and suggest recommendations for reading materials or behavioral exercises to be completed at home. Couples- and relationship-therapy that addresses broader partnership concerns may also help increase feelings of intimacy and desire.

DATING AFTER BREAST CANCER

If you were single when you received your cancer diagnosis, you may have put dating on hold. Now that you're done with treatment, you may be ready to meet potential new partners again. At the same time, the idea of diving back into the dating pool may fill you with anxiety. Many people who have had cancer worry that their medical history will scare away prospective partners. One study of online daters revealed that most people aren't deterred by a potential match who's had cancer. And experts agree that an experience with cancer shouldn't affect your chances of finding romance.

That's reassuring, but you still might have questions about navigating the dating scene.

When do I bring up cancer?
There's no one-size-fits-all answer to this question. It depends on your comfort level and your personality. If you're someone who likes to be upfront, you might refer to your cancer journey on your online dating profile. You might bring up the topic during your first conversation with a new match or your first in-person date. Other people prefer to wait until they've established a sense of comfort and trust. They would rather wait to see if there's potential for a longer-term relationship before discussing their cancer journey.

How much do I reveal?
This is another question that has no right or wrong answer. Some people are careful about how much they share at the start of a new relationship. Cancer may have affected your body, sexuality or fertility. It's understandable if you want to keep these issues private at first. You may feel more comfortable sharing information slowly, as a relationship progresses. Other people prefer to lay it all out there early. They want to gauge how the other person reacts and address concerns right away. The important thing is to be honest, at whatever pace works for you.

What should I say?
Before starting the conversation, take some time to plan it out. Think about how you'd like to bring up the topic and the words you want to use. You might even try practicing what you'll say out loud with a trusted friend.

As part of that conversation, consider sharing how it feels to reveal this information. Doing so will help someone better understand where you're coming from and how to respond. For example, you might say, "This is a little scary for me. I worry it will change how you see me." You can also deepen the conversation by asking open-ended questions such as, "How are you feeling about this?" or "Is there anything you're wondering about?"

Dealing with the fear of rejection
If you're scared to start dating again, you're not alone. Research shows that dating anxiety is common among breast cancer survivors. For example, in one study cisgender women who'd had breast cancer were more likely to be overly critical of their appearance, connecting how they looked to their sense of self-worth. For some cancer survivors, fear of rejection prevents them from dating at all.

If changes to your appearance are impacting your confidence, consider some of the body image boosters on page 138. Here are other strategies:

Practice self-compassion
Self-compassion is an attitude. It involves being kind to yourself, especially when you're caught up in harsh self-judgment. Self-compassion helps you remember that all people are imperfect, and that's OK. Try talking to yourself the way you'd talk to a treasured friend. Treating yourself this way may reduce some of your fears about dating.

Take the focus off dating
Having a romantic or sexual partner isn't the only way to find meaningful connections or to feel loved. Connect with friends and family in your social network. Engage in group activities you enjoy. Be open to new people, whether they be potential friends or a possible partner.

Talk to people going through what you're going through
Share your experiences and fears with trusted single friends or single members of a breast cancer support group. Just saying your worries out loud can often take away some of the anxiety. Hearing other people's stories can give you the confidence to try dating again.

Take dating one step at a time
Remove some of the pressure by shifting your expectations. Try to view dating as a chance to stretch yourself socially. If someone doesn't return your interest, don't assume cancer is to blame. Some matches aren't the right fit. That was true before you had cancer too.

Seek professional support
If anxiety about dating is freezing you in place, consider working with a licensed therapist, maybe one who is a sex therapist. These mental health professionals can help you work through your fears and gain the confidence to put yourself out there again.

10

Fertility and pregnancy

About 10% of breast cancer survivors are diagnosed at an age when they may have been looking forward to having children. If you're in this group, you may be wondering about whether it is possible and safe to have children after being treated for breast cancer, or whether your children might be affected by your history of breast cancer.

Or maybe pregnancy isn't on your radar yet — or you weren't planning on ever having kids — and you have questions about what birth control you can use, especially if you can no longer use hormone-based contraception.

Many people have concerns about their reproductive health as they enter the survivorship phase of their cancer journey. While statistics show that, on average, breast cancer survivors are 40% to 60% less likely to get pregnant than people who didn't have cancer, the good news is that many breast cancer survivors can and do get pregnant and deliver perfectly healthy babies. And for those looking to avoid pregnancy, there are safe and effective birth control options.

Sometimes it can feel as if topics such as fertility and contraception don't get the same attention as other aspects of survivorship. Addressing these topics is a crucial component of any survivorship plan and a key factor in your physical and emotional well-being. If no one on your health care team has discussed these topics with you yet, don't hesitate to start the conversation. This chapter covers the various aspects of reproductive health for survivors and can help lay the groundwork for you to have an in-depth discussion with your doctor or other members of your health care team.

CONTRACEPTION

Research has found that unplanned pregnancies among breast cancer survivors are common. The reason for that could involve any number of factors. There's a misconception among survivors that because breast cancer treatments can damage ovarian function and cause infertility, pregnancy is next to impossible.

Some survivors may also be under the impression that birth control methods such as intrauterine devices (IUDs) aren't safe for people who've had breast cancer, or that since they can't take hormonal birth control, there aren't many other options. Others may have received inadequate counseling to help them choose an effective contraceptive.

These scenarios may be why some survivors forgo birth control altogether or use a less effective approach, such as the withdrawal method, which involves withdrawing the penis from the vagina before ejaculation.

A recent study out of the United Kingdom highlights how crucial reproductive counseling is for breast cancer survivors. Researchers found that almost two-thirds of breast cancer survivors in the study weren't using birth control despite not wanting to get pregnant. Unfortunately, this puts survivors at an increased risk of an unplanned pregnancy. Unplanned pregnancies are problematic because many breast cancer survivors take endocrine therapy, such as tamoxifen, for five years or longer to prevent a recurrence. These medications can be harmful to a developing fetus.

Choosing contraception

Hormone-free contraceptives appear to be the safest choice for most breast cancer survivors and are what health care professionals typically recommend. Effective nonhormonal contraceptive options include:

- **Copper intrauterine devices** Paragard is an intrauterine device (IUD) that offers long-term birth control (up to 10 years) for premenopausal women. The device is a T-shaped plastic frame that's inserted into the uterus. It is 99% effective at preventing pregnancy. Copper wire coiled around the device produces an inflammatory reaction toxic to sperm and eggs, thus preventing pregnancy.
- **Double barrier method** This uses two forms of contraception: either a condom, female condom or diaphragm in conjunction with nonprescription spermicides such as nonoxynol-9 or a prescription vaginal contraceptive gel such as Phexxi. This method is 75% to 80% effective at preventing pregnancy.

- **Natural family planning** Natural family planning is a method of birth control that helps you predict when ovulation will happen based on observation of fertility indicators. It typically involves charting your temperature daily, tracking changes in cervical mucus and paying attention to other key fertility signs. This method is 75% to 80% effective at preventing pregnancy.
- **Sterilization** In women, you may have heard this referred to as tubal sterilization or "getting your tubes tied." In men, it's called a vasectomy. These surgical procedures stop eggs or sperm from traveling and are reserved for people who don't want children or are done having children. They're 99% effective at preventing pregnancy.

What about hormonal contraceptives?
Not as much is known about how hormonal methods of contraception — available in intrauterine devices, injectables and pills — may influence the risk of cancer progression or relapse in survivors. Hormonal birth control contains a combination of estrogen and progestin or progestin only that can encourage cancer growth.

Because of uncertainty regarding safety, health care professionals typically recommend that people with hormone receptor-positive breast cancer avoid these types of contraception.

In those who've had hormone receptor-negative breast cancer or a noninvasive form of breast cancer (ductal carcinoma in situ), hormonal birth control may be an option, but this is considered on a case by case basis and only after a thorough discussion about the risks and benefits with members of their health care team.

DO OVARIAN SUPPRESSION DRUGS WORK AS BIRTH CONTROL?

The short answer is no. Ovarian suppression drugs, also referred to as GnRH analogs, are sometimes prescribed as adjuvant endocrine therapy for premenopausal women with hormone receptor-positive breast cancer. Examples include leuprolide (Lupron) or goserelin (Zoladex). The goal in this case is to temporarily shut down the ovaries to decrease the level of estrogen in the body and reduce the risk of the cancer recurring. (These drugs can also be used to preserve fertility during cancer treatment.)

You might think that if you're taking medicine to shut down your ovaries — which stops menstruation in most women — that you wouldn't need birth control. But ovarian function may not be completely suppressed in some people, making pregnancy a possibility.

So don't assume you can't get pregnant if you're taking a GnRH analog. Talk to your primary care doctor about finding a nonhormonal contraceptive that works for you.

PREGNANCY AFTER CANCER

A planned pregnancy also is possible after breast cancer treatment. Studies have shown that about half of young women diagnosed with breast cancer express the desire to have children after treatment ends. But treatment such as chemotherapy, radiation, endocrine therapy and surgery can damage the ovaries or interrupt the menstrual cycle, triggering temporary or permanent infertility.

If you're like many survivors, concern about whether you can get pregnant is linked to a host of other concerns. You might also worry that your past treatments may directly impact a developing baby during pregnancy or create pregnancy complications. You may wonder whether the pregnancy itself increases your risk of breast cancer recurrence.

Common questions
Below are some of breast cancer survivors' most common questions regarding pregnancy after cancer treatment.

Can I get pregnant?
While there's no way to know for sure whether a successful pregnancy in an individual breast cancer survivor is possible, many women do get pregnant and deliver healthy babies after treatment. And it's not uncommon to conceive naturally. At the same time, multiple factors influence the likelihood of a successful pregnancy, including:

- Your age.
- The treatment you received (chemotherapy is known to lower the number of eggs a woman has).
- The protective measures used during treatment, such as temporarily suppressing ovarian function with medications such as leuprolide (Lupron) or goserelin (Zoladex).
- Your fertility status before treatment.
- The health of the sperm involved.
- The quantity and quality of your remaining eggs, also known as ovarian reserve.
- The frequency of your attempts to conceive.

Whether you used a fertility preservation technique before cancer treatment is also a factor. Preservation options include the following: freezing of your eggs, also called oocyte cryopreservation, for future fertilization and implantation; freezing an egg that's been fertilized by a partner or donor sperm, called embryo cryopreservation, for future implantation; or a procedure that involves removing part of, or the entire ovary for freezing. This last option is known as ovarian tissue cryopreservation. These procedures are performed before or during treatment and offer another way to get pregnant.

The risk of ovarian damage depends heavily on the type of cancer treatment received. For example, certain types of chemotherapy drugs can cause more damage than other kinds of treatment. A small study of breast cancer survivors who had undergone chemotherapy treatment found that up to three-quarters of the participants had their ovarian function return. However, this didn't guarantee the ability to get pregnant. Blood tests and imaging, such as ultrasound, can help your provider determine if your egg supply, or ovarian reserve, is healthy.

When is it safe to get pregnant?
Safely timing a pregnancy depends on many factors, whether you've had cancer or not. Fortunately, there doesn't appear to be an increased risk of cancer recurrence if conception happens soon after treatment ends, even among hormone receptor-positive breast cancer breast cancer survivors. Breastfeeding doesn't appear to raise the risk of recurrence either.

And recent studies suggest that getting pregnant within two years of treatment isn't harmful to the mother or baby, although there may be an increased

FERTILITY OPTIONS FOR MALE BREAST CANCER SURVIVORS

Men usually receive the same treatment as women for breast cancer and face infertility risks as well. Treatment can damage sperm, reduce sperm production and lower levels of hormones needed for reproduction, including testosterone. Male options for conception include:

- **Sperm banking** Male cancer patients may opt to bank their sperm before treatment. This simple process, also known as semen cryopreservation, involves freezing and storing sperm. Sperm can be frozen for an indefinite time.

- **Testicular sperm extraction** While cancer treatment can destroy the sperm in semen, sometimes there may still be healthy sperm in the testicles. Testicular sperm extraction involves removing small pieces of testicular tissue to look for healthy sperm cells, which can be used for in vitro fertilization (IVF).

risk of certain pregnancy complications, discussed in the next section.

If you're considering pregnancy, talk with your OB-GYN, oncologist or other members of your health care team. If you're on adjuvant endocrine therapy, you'll need to stop taking it and wait to conceive until the medication clears your system, since it can be harmful to a developing baby.

The good news here is that taking a break from endocrine therapy to have a baby does not increase the risk of cancer returning, according to a recent study of conception and pregnancy in young women who had early-stage hormone receptor-positive breast cancer. In addition, most of the women in the trial became pregnant and delivered healthy babies as desired — encouraging results for young breast cancer survivors who wish to start a family.

Will my past treatment affect my pregnancy and baby?
As in any pregnancy, prenatal care is critical to a healthy pregnancy and delivery. But there are some additional concerns for breast cancer survivors. On average, these pregnancies tend to result in infants with lower birth weight, smaller sizes for gestational age, greater likelihood of preterm delivery and greater chance of being delivered by Cesarean section.

Overall, though, most babies born to people who have undergone breast cancer treatment are healthy. They have no greater likelihood of genetic defects or postpartum health problems than those born without a maternal history of breast cancer. One exception is this: if you have a specific genetic mutation that increases cancer risk. In this case, your child has a 50% chance of inheriting this mutation. A genetic counselor can help you understand these hereditary risks. Ask your primary care doctor or oncologist for a referral if you need one.

FERTILITY OPTIONS

While conceiving naturally after breast cancer is possible, it's also possible to have difficulty doing so. If that's the case, you might consider using assisted reproductive technology (ART).

CAN I PREVENT MY BABY FROM INHERITING MY BREAST CANCER GENE?

Having a genetic variant such as BRCA1 and BRCA2 is understandably a concern when considering pregnancy. You may worry that you'll pass along this variant to your child. A child of someone carrying a genetic variant has a 50% risk of inheriting it. And because BRCA variants are dominant, it only takes one copy of a defective gene to increase the risk of breast cancer and other types of cancer, including ovarian, pancreatic and prostate cancers.

If your cancer is related to an inherited genetic variant, you may wish to speak with someone from your health care team or a genetic counselor about testing. Some people trying to conceive opt for preimplantation genetic testing (PGT). This technology can test for abnormalities in chromosomes, referred to as preimplantation genetic testing for aneuploidy (PGT-A), or for specific mutations linked to genetic diseases, known as preimplantation genetic testing for mutations (PGT-M). This testing is used when you attempt to conceive a child through IVF. Embryos are screened for congenital abnormalities. Those without these abnormalities are implanted into the uterus with hopes of resulting in pregnancy.

While this procedure eliminates the risk of your child carrying a cancer-causing gene, it may not be an option for everyone. Insurance may not cover the cost if it's being done solely to select a healthy embryo. And for some people, selecting which embryos are given a chance to develop and discarding extra embryos during PGT may not be acceptable from a religious or ethical standpoint.

In vitro fertilization (IVF)
IVF is the most common form of ART. It involves taking specific medicines to stimulate the ovaries to make eggs. If you started the IVF process prior to treatment, your eggs were collected and fertilized with your partner's or a donor's sperm in a laboratory. If fertilization is successful, the embryo or embryos can then be transferred into a uterus or frozen for later use.

When you're ready to become pregnant, an embryo is implanted, and you're given additional hormones to help sustain the pregnancy. In many cases, IVF isn't successful on the first attempt, and this process, also called a cycle, may need to be repeated.

Third-party reproduction options
Third-party reproduction options are another avenue to have children. This may involve:

Egg donation
If a survivor didn't store their eggs before treatment, eggs from another person might be an option. Eggs are typically from family, friends or anonymous donors. Donors are screened to ensure they have no serious health issues. The eggs then undergo the IVF process described earlier.

Gestational carrier
If a survivor's uterus isn't healthy enough to sustain a pregnancy, if the uterus has been removed or if it's unsafe to be pregnant, third-party reproduction (surrogacy) may be an option. This is when another person — the gestational carrier — carries the baby. Typically, what happens is that an embryo created from your eggs and sperm from your partner (or a donor) is transferred to a gestational carrier's uterus. The child will have your genes. No genes from the gestational carrier are passed

on to the child. Because laws for using another person (third-party) for pregnancy may vary depending on where you live, it's wise to contact a lawyer familiar with donor issues in your area for legal advice before proceeding.

Donor sperm
Male breast cancer survivors who didn't store sperm before starting treatment may wish to use donor sperm or sperm donated by a healthy man. The donor is usually anonymous, though the sperm is screened for diseases. A child conceived through donor sperm has the genes of the donor.

Adoption
Another option for starting a family is adopting an infant or child, with some potential qualifications. Some adoption agencies may require medical verification of your health. Others may make you wait for a certain period after completing treatment before you can adopt. Laws and adoption requirements differ from state to state and from country to country. A social worker or lawyer well-versed in adoptions can offer guidance on how to proceed.

You might also consider embryo adoption. This may be a choice for some people who can't use their eggs and don't have a partner or have a partner with male factor infertility. Previously created embryos from couples undergoing IVF are sometimes donated to embryo adoption agencies. These embryos can be legally adopted, and an embryo transfer can be performed to your uterus.

It's important to note that many of these options are expensive. Their costs may add to the financial burden many people with cancer already face. But there may be financial resources available to help with these costs. Ask a member of your health care team for referral to a social worker or financial counselor who can help you sort through your options.

COPING WITH EMOTIONS

Like cancer, infertility can have far-reaching effects, impacting your mental health, relationships and finances. Having to cope with both cancer and infertility can be especially challenging.

It's important to give yourself enough time to process your emotions and grieve the losses you feel. Although it can be difficult for people who haven't dealt with cancer and infertility to understand what you're going through, your loved ones no doubt will still want to offer you support. Keep the lines of communication open to your partner, family and friends to avoid isolating yourself. You may also want to enlist the help of a mental health professional or find a local support group where you can talk to people in similar circumstances, or both.

Feeling anger, loss and other emotions is entirely natural. Showing compassion for yourself can help you heal. So can time.

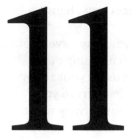

Family and friends

During your cancer treatment, some family and friends might have rallied around you. They might have provided invaluable support and adapted to your needs. Other people in your network might have withdrawn from you or avoided talking about your illness. And still others might have been a bit too nosy, asking questions you'd prefer not to answer. You've had to navigate it all as well as you could.

Now that you're in this next phase, you're navigating your relationships in a new way.

You might be wondering how to balance the expectations of your family and friends with your own needs as you recover from the physical and emotional effects of treatment. Friends and family often expect life to return to old rhythms and routines after treatment, not realizing that the experience of cancer can change a person.

And then there's the questions you may have about your social life. How do you restart friendships that may have faltered? If you want to focus on your recovery, is there a way to gracefully step back from your social circle? How can you protect your privacy while remaining open to the people in your life?

Chances are that you'll run into a few relationship conundrums over the coming weeks and months. Knowing what to expect can help you plan for those challenges and overcome them together.

EASING BACK INTO FAMILY LIFE

For some couples and families, cancer has a way of drawing them together. Previous arguments, disagreements and pet peeves seem to fade away in the face of the illness. You learn to treasure your moments with one another. Relationships can become stronger.

Illness places stress on relationships. If relationships were strained before cancer entered the picture, they may become even more strained now.

Even in the strongest of families, the period of recovery often comes with ups and downs. Getting back into the swing of things isn't always a smooth process. It can take time and effort to renegotiate your roles and find a new rhythm that works for you and your loved ones.

Common challenges
Cancer disrupts family life in big and small ways, creating unexpected challenges. Here are some common obstacles couples and families may face:

Big emotions
Your family members may have been laser focused on getting you through treatment. Like you, they were living day to day, taking life one step at a time. Now that active treatment is over, all the feelings, thoughts and fears they pushed aside may be hitting them hard. Your family may need time to process what they themselves experienced while you were in treatment. It can help to be aware that they may be dealing with some of the same thoughts and emotions you're working through.

Changed roles and responsibilities
If you were a take-charge kind of person before cancer, you might have found that during treatment your partner had to take over that role. Maybe you had to give up some of your responsibilities around the house or as an income provider to deal with treatment.

In turn, your partner might have picked up added responsibilities, such as making dinner, taking care of the children or working an extra job. Other family members, such as teenaged children, might also have pitched in to cover the responsibilities you used to handle. Deciding when and how to switch back to your old family routine — or create a new one — can be confusing and awkward.

Confusing expectations
Recovery doesn't always happen on the timeline you or your family expect. You might have assumed that everything would go back to normal right away. The problem is, you might not feel up to taking on all your former duties and routines. Your perspective and priorities might also have changed. Maybe you don't want the same duties and routines; maybe you want different ones.

If your recovery isn't going as well as you'd hoped, both you and your family might be frustrated.

> **"** It's important to be able to be vulnerable and authentic with family and friends. — L. K.

Sometimes you might feel pressured to do more than you can handle. It could seem as if all the support you experienced during treatment has vanished.

On the other hand, some loved ones may be overly attentive. You might find yourself being smothered with good intentions. Some family members might want to baby you and insist on doing things for you when no assistance is needed. They love you and want to help, but in fact they're too helpful.

Working as a team
It can be difficult juggling your recovery with your family's wants and needs. As in most situations, communication is key. Speaking openly with each other allows you to problem solve together and take everyone's perspective into account.

Some families find it helpful to schedule weekly or monthly meetings to address challenges that come up and to connect with one another. This can be a time to encourage honest communication about what each of you may be feeling. Sharing your thoughts and emotions in a calm and respectful way can help relieve tension and bring your family closer together.

Here are other ways to support one another and work together as a team:

Encourage patience
Sometimes it can feel like you're recovering at a snail's pace. You want to dive back into your old responsibilities but you're just not able to. Be sure to balance time to heal with time spent transitioning back to some

routines. Making space for recovery lessens your risk of injury and worsening fatigue. Try to take life one day at a time. As you continue to recover, you'll get to a place that feels comfortable.

Ask your family for their patience, too. Let them know when you need a break and when you're ready to return to an activity.

Be honest and specific
Some cancer survivors feel guilty asking for help when they've already received so much support during treatment. They think they should be able to go it alone now, but that might not be realistic.

If you aren't ready to take on all the responsibilities you had around the house before your cancer diagnosis, don't feel pressured to resume those duties too soon. But do tell your family what to expect so they aren't left wondering. Be specific about what you can and cannot tackle.

On the other end of the spectrum, some family members may insist on doing tasks you're perfectly capable of doing yourself. They might hover around you or pressure you to get more rest. This kind of overprotectiveness is well meaning but can be frustrating. Don't be afraid to speak up. Let your family know that you appreciate their care but that you're ready to take up your prior duties. Explain that these tasks can help you feel more normal and aid in your recovery.

Decide on your priorities
As a couple or a family, consider all the responsibilities of your household. What matters most to you? What can you put on hold for a while longer? Where can you temporarily lower your standards or ask for help?

Maybe you clean the shower a little less often or let the laundry pile up a little higher. Perhaps you ask if a friend or relative would be willing to pitch in with household tasks, such as doing yardwork, grocery shopping or preparing a few meals. Or, if it's feasible, you might pay for some of these services for a few weeks or months.

Express gratitude
Let your partner, children and other family members know that you appreciate the specific ways they've supported you. For example, if your children have taken on extra chores, acknowledge how much their contributions have meant to you in specific terms. Maybe their help allowed you to conserve your energy to attend a family event you otherwise could not have attended. As you're able to resume those chores, make sure your children understand that those responsibilities no longer rest on their shoulders.

Have fun together
Life isn't all about cancer, but sometimes that's hard to remember. Remind your family by engaging in activities that bring you all joy. Watch a movie that makes

---

" Many things in life remind us of our mortality. Of course, cancer does that. So does aging and other physical ills. My mother's recent death left me feeling almost as exposed as my cancer. And my daughter almost died, in an instant, in a freak accident. The best we can do is cultivate gratitude for each day we have and try to be nice people, and love those who love us. — P. W.

you laugh together. Go on a walk around the block. Play a board game or video game. Visit a zoo or museum.

Seek help
Coping with recovery may require skills that you and your family don't use on a daily basis. It's not only appropriate, but often wise, to seek help in the form of counseling.

A faith leader or licensed mental health professional can provide you and your family an outlet for discussing and working through feelings you might not express on your own. This person may also offer coping skills to help strengthen your relationships and work through disagreements.

SUPPORTING YOUR CHILDREN

Once treatment is over, your children might wonder why you aren't immediately back to your old self. If you can't yet participate in their lives as fully as you once did, they may silently worry they're to blame. They may also have questions about what your doctor is doing to keep you safe.

The instinct of most parents is to protect their children from difficult topics. But children do better when they're given information that's appropriate for their age and maturity level. Without accurate information they may misinterpret what's happening or make up theories that don't reflect reality. When you're willing to share facts and answer questions, children tend to be less fearful. Open communication also nurtures a sense of support, closeness and trust. They will be more willing to share openly with you in return.

Explain how your recovery may affect daily life

If recovery is going slowly, your physical and emotional resources may be low. Symptoms such as fatigue or pain can make it difficult to play with your children or engage the way you want to. Be honest about how your ongoing recovery might affect your children. Explain that as you're healing, you might not be able to participate in all the activities and events you used to. Reassure them that you are working to restore your abilities so you can participate. Tell them you love them and that you'll get stronger with time. This kind of conversation can prevent hurtful misunderstandings or feelings of isolation.

Explain what happens next

Let your children know that you'll continue to see your health care team for follow-up care. How much detail you go into will depend on your child. For example, you might tell a young child that you'll keep going to medical appointments to make sure you're healthy. Older children may benefit from a more in-depth conversation. They might want to know how and why your health care team is monitoring you. Be accurate in what you tell them and share your hope for the best outcome. Let them know you're in good hands and that your health care team is monitoring you closely.

Answer and ask questions

Kids take in what they're emotionally mature enough to understand. As they age, they might ask questions you've already answered. Or they may want additional information. Be prepared to answer their questions, even if you have to repeat yourself over the coming weeks, months and years.

You can also invite your children to share their thoughts and feelings by asking them questions. What would they like to know about your recovery or your follow-up care? Or do they feel that you're telling them the right amount of information, too little, too much? Are there any thoughts, feelings or questions they've been afraid to share with you?

These kinds of questions may be scary to ask at first. It can be hard to delve into your child's feelings, especially if some of them are negative. But your children may need you to get the conversation started, especially if they're afraid of burdening you with their thoughts or questions. Opening the lines of communication lets your child know it's okay to talk about what's going on inside of them. Explain that it's normal to have a range of feelings, even emotions like anger, sadness or resentment. Be a role model — share that you have these feelings too. You can also reassure them that it's safe to ask questions or tell you what's on their mind.

Pay attention

Keep tabs on how your children are behaving. Inform important adults in their lives about your illness and ask them to also keep tabs on behavior. Teachers, principals and school counselors can provide support and help your child cope. This helps form a strong support network for your child.

Noticeable changes, such as acting younger, becoming more clingy, withdrawing or having trouble in school, can indicate that a child is struggling. If you or other important adults notice a change in your child, ask your child how they're doing and if there are ways you or others can help them feel better. If the behavior changes last longer than a few weeks, consider talking to your child's doctor or nurse, school counselor or another mental health professional.

Spend extra time together

Your children crave time with you, and time is a powerful way to show your love. If you're still healing, choose low-key activities. Watch a silly TV show or read a book together. Play a card game or work on a jigsaw puzzle. Take a trip to a playground or go on a short walk. These kinds of experiences can help you reconnect and strengthen your bond.

Be kind to yourself

The healing process may put up a temporary roadblock when it comes to parenting. You may feel guilty taking time out to rest and relax as you recover. Remind yourself that self-care is the best way to replenish your physical and emotional reserves. The sooner you regain your strength and well-being, the sooner you'll be able to fully engage as a parent.

RECONNECTING WITH FRIENDS

Friendships sometimes deepen during a health crisis like a cancer diagnosis. During your treatment, your friends may have encircled you, lending their support in a variety of meaningful ways.

It's common, though, for some friendships to falter. Certain friends might be frightened by having someone so close to them develop a life-threatening illness. Your diagnosis might have brought up worries about their own health or painful memories of loss. Other friends might not know what to say or how to handle the situation, and they worry they'll accidentally upset you. Unsure how to respond, they may distance themselves. These reactions can be hurtful and leave you feeling isolated. It helps to keep in mind that your friends'

HOW DO I HELP MY CHILDREN MANAGE THEIR FEARS OF RECURRENCE?

The topic of cancer recurrence is tricky to navigate with children and teens. Many parents avoid the subject. For younger children, that might make sense. It may be appropriate to shield them from this complex topic until they're old enough to grasp it.

Preteens and teenagers often understand more about recurrence but may be afraid to bring up the subject. They might feel they should be strong for you and bottle up their fears. They also may sense you're hiding your own fears from them, which can cause them distress.

If your children ask questions, answer them as best as you can. Let them know that it's normal to have some fears and worries about the future. Talk with them about ways they might work through their feelings. Sometimes, just being close together without even talking is helpful in easing anxious thoughts. Give your child a long hug, snuggle on the couch or observe the outdoors together. Other helpful emotional outlets for your child might include drawing, writing in a journal or talking to a mental health professional.

reactions are usually driven by fears, such as worrying they'll say the wrong thing.

Before feelings of loneliness and isolation get you down, remember that you can take steps to nurture

TALKING TO FAMILY MEMBERS ABOUT THEIR CANCER RISK

As a cancer survivor, be aware that some of your relatives may be at greater risk of developing breast cancer themselves. This can include your parents, siblings and children. The risk increases if you have a gene mutation linked to breast cancer, such as BRCA1 or BRCA2.

If you've undergone genetic testing, share the results with your parents, siblings and adult children. Your genetic counselor can help you determine if additional family members should be informed. Providing loved ones with accurate information helps ensure that their health care teams recommend appropriate cancer screenings.

If your breast cancer is linked to a specific genetic variant, let family members know what that variant is. You might also suggest they meet with a genetic counselor, but avoid forcing the issue. Some cancer survivors share the information with extended family through a letter. Or they enlist a trusted family member to talk to the appropriate relatives. This information can cause fear, so it is important to include empowering actions family members can take to safeguard their health, such as screening and preventive surgeries.

If your children are under the age of 18, you might want to hold off on having this conversation. Genetic testing generally isn't recommended for minors, and most cancer screenings don't begin until adulthood. Follow your child's lead by answering questions as they arise.

> **"** At first, I tried to be everything everyone wanted me to be — strong, fun and courageous. Over time, I discovered who was still there when I was in the dark times. I let the people who would disappear just kind of drift away. I found that the people who were steady were also the most fun in the good times. — C.

relationships with friends. The first step is to acknowledge that most of these people care about you, and they each have their own way of reacting to your cancer. Here are some other tips for reconnecting with friends and repairing your relationships:

Start the conversation
Some people might want to ask how you're feeling, but they don't know what to say. Or maybe they think they'll upset you. Start the conversation yourself. Let people know that you welcome their questions. If you'd rather focus on other topics, explain that, too. Let friends know that you don't wish to talk about your cancer right now but would like to catch up on other things.

Ask for help when you need it
Some friends may take a big step back now that your treatment is complete. Be willing to ask for their support when you need it, even if it's just being there to talk. The people in your life might not realize that recovery can take time and that you could still use a helping hand. Friends feel good when they can support you.

Stay involved when you can

Some friends might not invite you to do things because they assume you aren't yet ready for social activities. Let these people know when you want to be included — or ask someone else to relay your message.

Know when to let go

Some people may continue to withdraw from you, and you'll have to let them go. Try not to expend a lot of emotional energy trying to patch up relationships that may not have been strong to begin with. Invest your time and energy in the friends who are closest to you.

Fill in the gaps with support groups

You'll have times when you feel that people who haven't had cancer don't understand what you're going through. Support groups can help meet the human need to feel understood. Discussing your feelings with other cancer survivors, whether in a support group in your community or online, may be helpful.

Choosing to step back

Some cancer survivors find it exhausting to spend a lot of time on various friendships while recovering from treatment. Instead, they might feel the need to invest their energy into healing themselves, spending time with family or getting back into other areas of their lives.

Whatever you feel is okay. It's okay to take the time you need for yourself. If friends reach out to you before you're ready, let them know you're still in recovery mode. Most people will understand and want to give you the space you need. Those friendships will still be there when you want to reconnect.

You may also be realizing that you prefer to let go of certain casual or less supportive friendships. That's okay, too. The cancer experience may have clarified which friendships mean the most to you.

Protecting your privacy
Some people ask a lot of questions — perhaps more than you're comfortable answering. It helps to decide ahead of time how you'll respond to such questions and what boundaries you want to set. You might say that you don't feel comfortable answering those questions. Or you might avoid the issue by changing the subject or redirecting the conversation.

On the other hand, you may welcome questions from trusted friends. It can be a relief to talk freely with someone who cares about you and shares in what you're going through. Even so, there may be days when cancer is the last thing you want to discuss. If that's the case, explain that although you've been open in the past, today you need a break from the topic.

A PERIOD OF ADJUSTMENT

The days, weeks and months after treatment are a time of adjustment — not only for you but for those close to you. As you move through this phase together, keep the channels of communication open by clarifying your limits, expressing your needs, and setting healthy boundaries. Your relationships will benefit, and so will you.

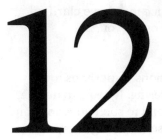

Work and money

An aspect of breast cancer that's not often talked about is the toll it can take on your career and finances. Almost half of breast cancer survivors are of working age when they're diagnosed. While some may be able to work through treatment, others reduce their work hours, take a leave of absence or leave the workforce entirely. In fact, breast cancer survivors are more likely to be unemployed than people who've never had cancer.

Chemotherapy and mastectomy — and all the side effects linked to these treatments — increase the odds of not returning to work. Some survivors may struggle if they have to return to a work environment that's not supportive or that discriminates against them. About half of breast cancer survivors are also dealing with the financial fallout from the disease, which you may hear referred to as financial toxicity. It's estimated that out-of-pocket medical debt for breast cancer survivors can be more than $10,000 during the first year after diagnosis alone.

While the professional and financial obstacles following a breast cancer diagnosis can be daunting, there's good news: most breast cancer survivors who aren't retirement age do return to the workforce. For many, this means a return to some normalcy and another step forward to a life beyond breast cancer. And there are resources available to help you navigate the financial side of breast cancer — if you know where to look and whom to ask.

RETURNING TO WORK

Before you finished treatment, perhaps you were determined to go back to your job and settle into your prediagnosis work routine once treatment was over. However, as you may be discovering, it's not always that simple. Many survivors struggle with reentering the workforce and picking up where they left off.

Reasons for reluctance
There are several reasons why people might feel reluctant to return to work after finishing breast cancer treatment. See if any of the following sound familiar.

You have a new perspective
Sometimes it's hard to return to your old career because you are reevaluating your priorities. Your job may not seem as fulfilling or meaningful as it once did. You might feel this is the time to try something new.

> " Physically I was exhausted, but emotionally and spiritually I was renewed and exhilarated. I promised to never take my life for granted again. I put my store up for sale, started a new job that meant way less stress in my life. I have never looked back, nor have I broken that promise to myself. — C.

You have lingering limitations
Some people find they need to pivot to a new career because of lingering side effects of treatment that make former responsibilities too difficult. Fatigue, for example, is a commonly reported residual side effect of cancer treatment. Brain fog is another. You may have trouble remembering minutiae, focusing on long-term projects, or juggling long meetings and busy work. You also might have lymphedema, which can make physically demanding jobs challenging to perform, or you might have limited range of motion because of your mastectomy, radiation or both.

You're worried about how limitations will affect you
You're concerned that your work performance won't be as good as before you were diagnosed. You're afraid you won't be able to handle stress or workload the way you used to. These can be reasonable fears if you still have residual side effects from treatment.

You're self-conscious
You might be worried about how you look, from hair in an awkward regrowth stage to feeling self-conscious about the loss of your breast or breasts, or the arm bandages used to treat your lymphedema.

Work support is lacking

Sometimes, an employer may not understand your difficulties or may be inflexible with specific accommodations, such as limited work hours or a work-from-home arrangement. Your boss may even doubt you can still do your job. Coworkers may be resentful that you get certain accommodations, like different work hours.

Getting back into the swing of things

Often, the simple act of acknowledging the obstacles you face and understanding how they affect you can help you get a clearer picture of how you want to proceed in your professional journey.

If you've decided it's time to reenter the workforce, your first practical step is to get your health care team's OK. If you have been on short- or long-term disability, make sure you and your care team have completed the paperwork necessary for your return to work.

Next, set up a meeting with your supervisor or human resources representative to discuss returning to work and any accommodations you may need. Accommodations include any change or adjustment made when you have a disability that makes it easier to do your job. Accommodations are covered under the Americans with Disabilities Act, or ADA (see more about the ADA later in this chapter). Review your employer's policies to understand their process for requesting accommodations. According to the ADA, you do not have to use the words "reasonable accommodation" in your request or meeting.

Accommodations can include:

- **A schedule adjustment** You may want to start by working part-time to see how things go or reworking your schedule so you can more easily accommodate follow-up medical appointments. In addition, you may want to ask your supervisor or human resources department whether you can take regularly scheduled breaks to take medication or deal with fatigue.

- **Working from home** If your job allows, telecommuting or working from home at least some of the time may help to minimize fatigue around commuting or anxiety around fitting back into the workplace.
- **Sharing tasks** Until you're ready for full-time work, ask if some of your nonessential tasks can be temporarily redistributed among coworkers or if you can work together with coworkers on big projects.
- **Performing a different job** If your hours change or you're unable to perform essential tasks in your old job, ask if there's a suitable job you can do instead temporarily.

If you find yourself struggling, reach out to your supervisor or human resources department to make them aware of the situation and to see if any additional accommodations can be made. For some, work may not be an option until treatment symptoms subside.

In some cases, you may need to provide documentation of your current limitations to support your requested accommodations or to extend your disability leave. Discuss with your primary care team whether you need to consult with a physical or occupational therapist related to this documentation.

Dealing with coworkers

Coworkers who support a return to work give survivors confidence that they can successfully transition back to their jobs. However, it's up to you how much you're willing to share about your diagnosis and treatment with your coworkers (and what kind of support you would like). Many survivors prefer that their coworkers treat them the same as they did before diagnosis.

It's normal to feel stress about how to answer coworkers' questions once you return. You'll likely find most coworkers supportive and ready to welcome you back. But be prepared for a wide range of questions and reactions, from empathy and understanding to resentment for having had to carry a bigger workload in your absence. Some may ask blunt questions, such as about your hair or lymphedema bandage, that you may not want to answer.

Preparing for these questions regarding how you look, feel and the time you've been gone can minimize stress. It may be helpful to practice with a close friend or family member how you'll answer these questions. Remember, this is your narrative, and you can choose when and how much you share with coworkers. If you're regularly being made to feel uncomfortable, don't hesitate to bring it up with your supervisor or human resources department.

In some cases, it may be beneficial for an employer to hold informational meetings on employment topics such as the ADA and the workplace and reasonable accommodations to ensure that everyone understands their protections. This can help avoid misconceptions that workers using ADA protections are getting special treatment.

Taking time for yourself
Don't forget to take care of yourself. Eating well, exercising regularly and getting enough sleep can help you maximize your confidence and productivity. You may find it helpful to participate in a rehabilitation program to treat cancer-related side effects, or you might want to join a local support group that helps you connect with other survivors who understand what you're going

through. See Chapters 3 and 4 for strategies on staying healthy and coping with treatment side effects.

Supportive family members can also be a great help as you go back to work. Ask your loved ones if they are willing to take on more responsibilities at home so that you can focus more on transitioning back to work.

Returning to work is a significant adjustment, and you may need extra time before you can get back to a regular schedule. Give yourself grace. Though you may feel pressure to get back to your job, returning before you're fully ready can leave you struggling and your work suffering. Don't feel guilty about taking your time in this next stage of recovery. Everyone benefits when you're at your strongest.

FINANCES IN SURVIVORSHIP

For many people, decisions about work and career hinge not just on personal preferences but financial need. Most people understand that cancer care is costly. But until it happens to you, it's hard to fathom just how draining treatment can be on personal finances.

It's not uncommon for survivors to have outstanding bills from surgeries, chemotherapy or radiation. Some survivors travel long distances or use out-of-network healthcare providers to get the care they feel is best.

Long-term therapies, such as those used to prevent breast cancer recurrence and those used to treat metastatic disease, can prolong financial problems. And young survivors are particularly likely to have gaps in their insurance or no insurance at all.

Financial toxicity goes beyond monetary terms. It also refers to the mental health burden that can come with struggling economically, including worrying about

> Breast cancer not only affects you physically, but mentally and emotionally as well. And then there are the financial challenges that come from the cost of treatment, loss of pay due to time off for treatment or treatment related illness, lack of adequate insurance, or for some, lack of any kind of insurance. There are so many resources available to help patients who need financial support. At our nonprofit supporting single mothers with advanced breast cancer, I recommend that a patient speak to their care team about options and resources as soon as possible so they can become familiar with their options from the onset. — R. L.

money and curtailing basics, such as food or medicine, to pay your medical bills.

If you're facing financial difficulties because of your cancer care, it's important to get help. Knowing what resources are available to you can help you make better work and life decisions in the long run.

First steps

First off, tell someone on your cancer care team as soon as possible. Your team will want to know whether you're having trouble paying for things like nonmedical expenses or copays for office visits or medication, all of which can affect whether you follow your survivorship plan as prescribed.

Most cancer clinics have staff on hand to talk to you about finances related to cancer treatment, including social workers, case managers, financial counselors and atient navigators. Even if you're far from where you received treatment, you may be able to receive help through telehealth or over the phone. You can also reach out to your primary care team or insurance company for help finding the right resources. In addition, check out the list of resources on page 209 at the end of this book.

Social workers, case managers, financial counselors and patient navigators can do the following:

- Communicate with billing offices. You may be able to address outstanding bills with payment plans and reduced rates.
- Assist you in finding alternative financial resources, including from government, nonprofit and charitable institutions. Programs sponsored by these organizations may help pay for breast cancer survivors' bills, including noncancer-related expenses such as rent, utility bills and living expenses.
- Help you assess your current insurance and whether you're eligible for other programs, such as Medicare and Medicaid. If you're uninsured, a navigator could help you find insurance.
- Work with you to save on medications. (See "Saving on medications" on the next page.)

If you're undergoing treatment for recurrence or metastatic cancer, connecting with a social worker and patient navigator can allow you to access resources that are sometimes only available to patients going through active treatment.

Handling finances can often feel overwhelming. Consider asking a trusted family member or friend who is capable in this area for help keeping track of bills, insurance claims and key contacts. Such an arrangement may benefit both of you, allowing your loved one to help in a specific way and you to have greater peace of mind.

SAVING ON MEDICATIONS

The cost of medication can be a burden on cancer survivors. Some may consider skipping a dose or saving doses for later. However, this can impact the effectiveness of treatment. To help curb the cost of medication safely:

- Ask your health care provider whether lower-cost generic medications are available instead of name-brand. Sometimes taking a different form of the drug, such as a pill, is cheaper than other forms of medication.
- Look into discount drug programs. Nonprofits such as needymeds.org and drug companies often have programs that help pay for prescription drugs. A social worker or your cancer care team should be able to help you with this resource.
- Consult your insurance about using a mail-order pharmacy. Many insurance companies offer the option of purchasing medications by mail, and it may be cheaper than buying from your local pharmacy.
- Check with your insurance regarding which pharmacies are in-network. Using an in-network pharmacy will provide lower out-of-pocket costs for medications.

Paying for medical costs

Many people receive health insurance through their employer or a government-sponsored program, such as Medicare or Medicaid. However, not all do. You can purchase health insurance on the health insurance marketplace if you don't qualify for government programs.

The 2010 Patient Protection and Affordable Care Act (ACA) prohibits insurers from discriminating against you based on your health history and preexisting conditions when applying for primary insurance. However, health restrictions for some policies, such as Medicare supplementals, may still apply. For more information, visit healthcare.gov or call 800-318-2596 (TTY: 855-889-4325).

Some types of insurance may be a better fit for your needs.

Private insurance

Two of the most common types of private insurance include health maintenance organizations, or HMOs, and preferred provider organizations (PPOs). HMOs cover medical costs within a specific network of providers, but choices for providers are limited. PPOs tend to have a larger pool of healthcare providers to choose from compared to HMOs and may cover out-of-network providers, too. If you're unsure of your coverage or potential out-of-pocket costs at any time, call the number on the back of your card.

How to purchase insurance You can enroll in the health insurance marketplace's plans during the open enrollment period. (Check healthcare.gov for dates.) If you're in need of an insurance plan outside of the enrollment period, you may still qualify in special circumstances, such as having a child, getting married, losing health care coverage or experiencing some other life change. You can enroll at any time if you qualify for Medicaid or the Child Health Insurance Program (CHIP). In some cases, the health insurance marketplace may redirect you to your state's own insurance site.

Government-sponsored insurance
Federal health insurance options include Medicare (for those 65 and older and Americans that have been certified disabled by the Social Security Administration for a minimum of 2 years) and Medicaid (for younger people, usually based on low income).

Medicare has multiple parts covering care aspects such as skilled nursing, hospice, physical and occupational therapy, prescription medications and some medical supplies. Medicare parts A and B cover 80% of medical costs. Without additional coverage, you are responsible for the remaining 20% of the costs.

Federal and state governments fund Medicaid. Since each state has its own program, eligibility and services differ from state to state. In general, the program covers individuals below a certain level of income and those with a disability. In some states, Medicaid is available to help pay for breast cancer-related treatments or screenings and is not based on income. Speak with your oncology team or with your cancer center's financial navigator, nurse navigator or social worker for guidance on federal and state programs for which you may qualify.

How to sign up for Medicare or Medicaid The following sites can assist you in determining your eligibility or explaining how to apply.
- Medicaid: medicaid.gov
- Medicare: medicare.gov
- Affordable Care Act: healthcare.gov

The State Health Insurance Assistance Program (shiphelp.org) offers local, unbiased, one-on-one help for reviewing Medicare plan options, coverage, eligibility and other issues.

Social Security Disability Insurance

If you've paid into the Social Security Disability Insurance (SSDI) program through your job and you find yourself disabled because of cancer treatment, you and your spouse and children may be eligible for SSDI benefits. It's not uncommon to get turned down for SSDI when you first apply, and not all cancer diagnoses qualify for SSDI. Many times, appeals of the decision are successful, but you must meet Social Security's strict definition of disabled, which is detailed in their Social Security "Blue Book Disability Evaluation Under Social Security" (ssa.gov/disability/professionals /bluebook).

Certain cancer diagnoses, such as metastatic breast cancer, are called "Compassionate Allowance Conditions" by the Social Security Administration. Approval may be expedited if you currently have cancer that's identified on the Compassionate Allowance list and you meet specific criteria.

For those who received SSDI benefits during treatment and want to return to work, Social Security offers a free program called Ticket to Work. This provides support while you try to return to work. During a return-to-work trial period, you will get disability benefits. Visit choosework.ssa.gov for more info, or call 866-968-7842 or your local Social Security office.

How to apply for SSDI Consider talking with a financial navigator, nurse navigator or social worker to better understand eligibility and the process of applying for SSDI. You can apply online at ssa.gov/benefits/disability /apply or by calling 800-772-1213 (TTY: 800-325-0778). You can also reach out to your local SSA office by phone or in person. If you're not eligible for SSDI, a program called Supplemental Security Income (SSI) may be an option. For more information, visit ssa.gov.

Other ways to pay
Additional resources that may help you cover medical costs include:

Supplemental insurance
If you purchased supplemental insurance prior to your cancer diagnosis, review the policies to determine how they may be able to help you now. Supplemental insurance can help pay for cancer care costs not covered by regular insurance and, in some cases, lost wages if you can't work. Examples of supplemental insurance include specialized plans that cover disability, hospital stays or long-term care. Supplemental insurance is often subject to restrictions such as preexisting conditions and may not be available to purchase after a diagnosis.

Savings accounts
If you have a flexible savings account (FSA) or health savings accounts (HSA) — bank accounts that allow you to put money away for out-of-pocket medical expenses, usually with tax benefits — these funds can help you pay for a variety of costs, if they qualify as medical expenses. FSAs and HSAs are usually offered through employers and private insurance.

Nonprofits
The National Cancer Institute maintains a database of organizations that provide a wide range of resources and allows you to tailor search results to your specific needs. Visit supportorgs.cancer.gov or call 800-4-CANCER. Additional resources include the Cancer

financial Assistance Coalition (cancerfac.org), CancerCare (cancercare.org) and Triage Cancer (triage-cancer.org).

Tax benefits
In some cases, health care costs can be claimed on your income taxes. For example, you may be able to deduct the costs associated with traveling to and from your doctor appointments. Ask your tax preparer if this option would benefit you.

KNOW YOUR RIGHTS

Cancer survivors can and do face discrimination in the workplace, so it's essential to know what protections are available. If you're facing problems at work, be sure to keep all correspondence you have around the issues you're experiencing. Make a running list of whom you've communicated with in case you run into legal issues.

Americans with Disabilities Act
While a history of cancer doesn't automatically qualify you for protection under the Americans with Disabilities Act (ADA), the law does protect people who have long-term disabilities because of cancer. A disability may be obvious, such as a limited range of motion following a mastectomy or arm swelling because of lymphedema. But some are less apparent, such as problems with cognition stemming from treatment. If you struggle with day-to-day activities or have health problems involving other parts of your body because of your cancer treatment — such as the brain, respiratory system or nervous system — you may qualify for

protection under the ADA. Each ADA case is looked at individually.

Under the ADA, an employer with 15 or more employees in the private sector, as well as state and local governments, must provide certain protections to their employees. Federal workers aren't covered by the ADA but have their own protections. The ADA makes it illegal to pay you less, deny you leave or fire you because you had cancer or a disability that prevents you from performing nonessential duties. You can't be denied a promotion because of your cancer. If you've asked for protection under the ADA, an employer can't retaliate against you. Your family members are also protected if their employer tries to terminate their employment because of your cancer.

The ADA doesn't protect in all instances. You can still be let go for legitimate reasons — for example, the company has a round of layoffs. You must also be qualified to perform the job and its essential duties, with or without reasonable accommodation. Sometimes, an employer can prove that accommodation would be too expensive or difficult to make.

To get reasonable accommodation, you need to ask for it. You may already have some suggestions in mind for accommodations. For example, you may already know you'll be too fatigued to commute each day to the office. Instead, you might propose that you work from home for the first six months to a year or work from home three days a week.

Some survivors looking for new employment after treatment are concerned that their history of cancer will come up during the interview process and that this might reduce their likelihood of being hired. You're not required to disclose that you had cancer, although some survivors do because they know they will need an accommodation. However, you're not obligated to discuss your disability until you ask for accommodation.

The ADA dictates which questions can and can't be asked during the various stages of the hiring process. For example, during your first interview, a potential employer can't ask if you've ever had cancer, what treatments you had or the type or severity of your disability. An employer can ask if you can perform the job and if you may need accommodations. Later in the process, an employer can ask for documentation from your health care team stating that you can perform the job safely.

Because the ADA can be complicated, reach out to a disability advocate or a vocational rehabilitation counselor. Such a person can help you with legal questions about your job. You may also want to reach out to the Job Accommodation Network at 800-526-7234 or askjan.org/media/Cancer. Additional legal resources can be found at Triage Cancer (triagecancer.org) and the Cancer Legal Resource Center (thedrlc.org/cancer).

If you think you're being discriminated against, file a complaint with the Equal Employment Opportunity Commission (EEOC) by calling 800-669-4000 or visiting ada.gov.

The Family and Medical Leave Act (FMLA)
Many cancer survivors are already familiar with this law, which grants employees at workplaces with at least 50 employees up to 12 weeks of unpaid time off for health issues. If you didn't use all 12 weeks during treatment, you might be able to use leave now for medical reasons. FMLA leave can be taken in days or even hours. If a family member is your caregiver during treatment, that family member can ask their employer if they are eligible for FMLA benefits. For more

information, visit the U.S. Department of Labor's
website (dol.gov).

The Genetic Information Nondiscrimination Act
Genetic testing allows health care teams to identify
predispositions to genetic disorders, including those
that cause breast cancer. However, some people avoid
testing because they're fearful the results could be used
against them, especially by health insurers and employers. The Genetic Information Nondiscrimination Act of
2008 (GINA) prohibits health insurers from discriminating against customers based on genetic information.
This piggybacks on the Health Insurance Portability
and Accountability Act (HIPAA) of 1996, which makes it
illegal for plans and insurers to label someone as having
a preexisting condition based on genetic information.

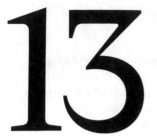

For partners

Caring for someone during cancer treatment is an intensely emotional time. Profound feelings of stress, anxiety and concern about your partner's health may have dominated your thoughts. You may have had to adjust your work life and other responsibilities to accommodate the demands of treatment. You may have had to take on your partner's duties around the house and elsewhere. You may have lost sleep, eaten poorly and not had time for exercise or social activities.

You may also be coping with feelings of grief and loss — having to let go of previous certainties about the direction your life was headed, plans you and your partner had, and even your daily routine. Life likely won't ever be the same again but you may feel guilty about mourning this kind of loss openly. You may also have feelings of frustration at changes in your relationship with your partner — emotionally, mentally and physically. It's not uncommon for caregivers to feel a degree of resentment toward their partners, for example, or to feel robbed of time or opportunities because of the cancer.

For many people, these personal costs are worth the value of supporting and caring for your loved one as they go through treatment. But as treatment ends or enters a new direction, it can take some time to adjust. What do you do now? How do you handle this new phase? Are you even the same person still? Is your relationship with your partner the same as it was before?

As the two of you come to grips with the situation and try to get your emotions in sync, you may be tested in new ways. You may need to make short-term and long-term adjustments in multiple areas of your lives. There will be good days, and there will be bad days. But be confident that you've made it this far and that you will have what it takes to move forward, one step at a time.

GIVE YOURSELF TIME

The end of intensive treatment often brings feelings of relief, but it can also bring concerns about cancer recurrence and lingering side effects, and even feelings of emptiness after spending so much time pursuing medical treatment goals and caring for your partner. Depending on the course of treatment, some caregivers may experience symptoms of trauma, such as distressing and unwanted memories. It's not uncommon for all parties involved to have both positive and negative thoughts about ending treatment.

Some people may feel, or may be pressured to feel, that they should be able to revert quickly to previous routines and that everything should go back to "normal." But treatment can have long lasting effects and, in some cases, may not be completely over.

It's important to give yourself time to process what you've been through. Allow yourself to feel what you feel, even if it feels strange or even "unacceptable." It's OK to grieve your losses. Allow these emotions to flow through. Make space for you and your partner to process the transition to survivorship in your own way.

TAKE CARE OF YOURSELF

When caring for someone else, it can be easy to become so focused on the needs of your loved one that you forget or ignore your own basic needs. But the results of doing so can lead to major problems. Caregivers often become frustrated, run-down and potentially burned out. Burnout is a state of emotional and physical exhaustion that often ends with the caregiver giving up his or her duties all together. Now that some of the demands of treatment have lifted, take time for yourself.

Address your physical needs

To give your loved one the best possible support, *you* need to be in good shape. During active treatment, you may have been so consumed with caring for your loved one, your home, your family and your job that you put yourself last. Now it's time to recuperate. This means making time to eat well, get enough sleep, engage in regular exercise and do things you enjoy. It's tempting to forgo these healthy habits, but carving out the time and help necessary to do so can lead to a better quality of life for you and your loved one.

WHEN YOU'RE A CAREGIVER BUT NOT A PARTNER

Breast cancer impacts not just the person with the disease but also the person's caregivers. Maybe you've been caring for a parent, sibling, relative or friend during their breast cancer treatment. You may have been there every day, accompanying your loved one to medical appointments and helping them at home. Or maybe you've been offering support remotely, working with your loved one's cancer care team, family members, friends and neighbors to coordinate care from afar. The National Cancer Institute defines a caregiver as anyone who helps another through diagnosis and treatment of cancer.

Caregivers are sometimes referred to as "invisible patients" because their health also is affected by the illness of those they care for. If you've been caring for someone throughout their breast cancer treatment, you may be looking at the next phase after active treatment with any number of mixed feelings — relief that surgery, chemo, radiation and other intense treatments are behind you but also uncertainty about what lies ahead.

This chapter is written primarily for partners of people with breast cancer, but anyone in a caregiver role may find portions of it helpful. Don't feel limited to this chapter, either. Other chapters in this book cover topics such as side effects of cancer treatment, talking with family and friends, and financial issues — all of which offer important information for caregivers as well as those who've gone through treatment.

" I had the very unfortunate opportunity to deal with my mother being diagnosed with stage 4 metastatic breast cancer and my 26-year-old (newlywed) daughter also being diagnosed with stage 1 breast cancer shortly after that. That was the scariest and most stressful thing that I've ever dealt with and if I didn't have a relationship with God, I wouldn't have made it.

It's very important to take care of the loved one that is battling this disease but you also have to take care of yourself. Taking time to wind down and decompress is important. I have experienced so many different emotions during this journey but the one that I experienced the most is thankfulness. I am so thankful that God healed my daughter and has allowed my mom (now 82 years old) to continue to live a good life. If I had to choose three words to describe this experience, I'd say, 'It is well.' — P. D.

Address your psychological needs

Good mental health is not just the absence of symptoms such as depression, anxiety and chronic stress. It means feeling satisfied with your life and fulfilled in what you're doing. Psychologists talk about three basic psychological needs that everyone has:

- **Freedom of will** This is the ability to make your choices your own. You do things because you want to and you believe in the worth of your actions, not because of pressure from others or to avoid conflict. Fulfilling this need — creating mental space to care for your partner because you want to and view it as important — creates a sense of integrity, where your actions are aligned with your values.

- **Relatedness** This is the feeling of warmth and care toward others, of mutual belonging, of supporting and being supported. Look for ways to connect with your partner and perhaps with others who have gone through similar experiences. Leaving this need unfulfilled results in feelings of isolation and loneliness.

- **Competence** This need is fulfilled when you engage in activities, and you experience opportunities for using and expanding your skills. You feel effective and confident. Make sure you have the information you need from your health care team so that you can feel confident in caring for your loved one in the best way.

Research suggests that for caregivers, focusing on these basic psychological needs can help bring out the positive aspects of caring for a loved one during illness and create better quality of life for the caregiver.

As you and your loved one move into the survivorship phase of the cancer journey, it may help to understand the options that are available to you so that you can freely make informed decisions. Support each other in your goals and priorities, and provide positive feedback on the activities and tasks you both choose to do. It can also help to share support with others who are in similar situations. Fulfillment of these needs can lead to high-quality motivation and purpose, which can increase long-term well-being, thriving and personal growth.

Integrate mindfulness

Mindfulness is a meditative-type tool that you can use anywhere, anytime to relieve stress, increase contentment and renew purpose. It's a systematic way of training your brain to be completely present in the moment, without judging and without relying on previous assumptions. Studies show that mindfulness-based stress reduction can help reduce caregiver stress and depression. It can also help you as a caregiver develop a deeper awareness of your reactions to your loved one's behaviors, as well as the emotional distance needed to adapt your responses accordingly.

Rediscover what makes you happy

After putting your all into caregiving, it's likely become a major part of your identity. If your partner is well on the way to recovery, you may find that you're not needed as much as you were before. It can be tough to let go of that sense of being the main one in charge. Try not to take it too personally. Instead, use your new free time and energy to rediscover your interests and hobbies, to catch up with close friends and to find new pleasures. By allowing for a bit of separation between you and your partner, you'll be able to come back with renewed appreciation for each other and fresh topics to discuss and interests to share.

Don't be a prisoner of fear

Cancer can make you confront the mortality of someone you love, and this can have profound effects. It may leave you feeling on edge, constantly on the alert for signs or symptoms of recurrence. You may feel a deep need to guard your feelings and avoid future pain by being hyperalert to any sign of bad news — always prepared and always vigilant. But constant worry about what lies ahead won't reduce your partner's risk. And it may make it more difficult to enjoy life as it is now.

One of the biggest challenges of survivorship is letting go of fear and uncertainty. But doing so can help you live a richer and more fulfilling life with your partner, one that is fully grounded in the present and that allows you to create positive memories you can carry with you forever.

Explore spirituality

For many people, religion and spirituality offer an important way to find meaning, hope and even joy amid the often-harsh realities of dealing with cancer.

Researchers have found that greater levels of religion and spirituality tend to be associated with better self-reported physical, mental and social health. Feelings of reverence, peacefulness and purpose can improve physical symptoms, such as fatigue and pain; reduce feelings of anxiety and depression; and improve the quality of relationships and social involvement.

Cancer also may raise doubts about core spiritual beliefs and bring up unanswered questions about why people suffer. Feelings of vulnerability, anger and betrayal — all very common — may lead you to question values or traditions you once thought unshakeable. Authentic experiences of religion and spirituality don't preclude struggling with why bad things happen.

One thing for sure is that a person's spirituality can change and evolve throughout life's journey. Even if it's an aspect of yourself that you haven't explored much in the past, it's never too late to do so. Here are some thoughts on how to get started.

- **Reflect** Spirituality is closely linked to self-discovery. When you have quiet time, think about yourself and the path your life has taken so far. What are the things that have truly mattered? What's important to you now? Many people use prayer or meditation to help them reflect on their inner lives.

- **Allow for struggle** Give yourself permission to wrestle with questions about meaning and existence or to leave them unanswered for a while. Often, that's how we grow and move toward spiritual wholeness.

- **Find beauty** Beauty has a long history of association with transcendence. Natural beauty in particular can inspire awe and reverence. A work of art may effectively capture what words fail to express about the human experience. Beauty can be found in simple things too, such as a piece of fruit or in the way light shines through a window. When you see something beautiful, let yourself experience it with all of your senses.

- **Connect** Sometimes, the most beautiful things in life are our relationships with others. To love and be loved, to belong and to cherish — these are certainly some of the most transcendent expressions of spirituality. Take every opportunity to turn toward your loved one. Find ways to enjoy each other's lives. Commit to comforting and supporting each other, even in the midst of struggle.

- **Seek help** You may wish to seek out spiritual resources in your community, such as a minister, priest, rabbi, imam or spiritual adviser who can talk with you about the issues that concern you. Many hospitals have chaplains and counselors who can help you address the psychological, emotional and spiritual aspects of dealing with cancer.

STAY SUPPORTIVE OF EACH OTHER

Importantly, support doesn't stop once treatment is over. Now more than ever, it's important to lean on each other. Chances are your partner is also feeling lost in the shuffle, and perhaps even abandoned now that medical appointments are spaced further apart and the near-daily support of the cancer care team is somewhat removed. Reading the other chapters in this book can help you understand a bit more what your partner may be going through.

It's likely that your loved one was given a follow-up care or survivorship plan (see page 23). It may help you to be familiar with the details of the plan, so that you can be supportive of next steps and of your partner's choices. Attend follow-up appointments together, if possible, especially at first or when tests are inconclusive. Doing this together will help you remember important information and provide each other with moral support.

Keep listening. Each person's experience of cancer is unique, so be open to what your loved one is feeling. Know that it's not your job to fix everything, but that it is important to be there, to validate your partner's feelings, and to offer reassurance of your love and support.

Discuss respective roles and responsibilities openly and honestly. Your partner may not be able to resume previously held duties, such as cooking or paying the bills, right away or even for a while. It may take some trial and error to establish a functional routine for the way things are now.

Sex with your partner is also likely to be different now than it was before the cancer diagnosis. Treatment may have changed your partner's self-image and libido, as well as caused physical changes that may affect your sexual relationship. Being patient and supportive of your partner's needs can deepen your connection and create more avenues for intimacy. See Chapter 9 for more on sexual intimacy.

> My wife Mary had three surgeries within two years. The first surgery was a bariatric sleeve operation, done to lose weight in preparation for a spinal surgery. Just before her spinal surgery, she was diagnosed with breast cancer. Mary and the doctors decided to do the spinal surgery first. Later, she underwent a double mastectomy and went flat without reconstruction.

In caring for her, I try to keep my mind open to her inner struggles and be more attentive to her needs. I keep quiet about my opinions regarding her pain and the loss of her breasts. I keep buying her flowers. I use her favorite creams to rub her back wounds. I make high-protein meals, vacuum, mop, make the bed and make sure the shower is equipped for her needs. One doesn't stay married for 52 years with all luck. There's also sacrificing, apologizing, forgiving, rebuilding a rebudding love, accepting her new body, and taking time for each other — yes, even a date night that I am lousy at.

Weight loss played a big role, too. My wife lost 80 pounds through bariatric surgery and I lost over 100 pounds through weight-loss medications. We are in our late 70s. If not for the significant weight loss, learning to eat better and daily exercise, my role as a caregiver would have been enormously more difficult. The benefits for myself as a caregiver and for Mary as a breast cancer patient were essential in sustaining our health, emotions and stamina during the healing process. — F. W.

Keep in mind that sometimes things can and will go wrong; be patient with yourself. Try to learn from mistakes, using them as opportunities to refocus your lens on life and come up with new, maybe even better, ways of doing things.

MOVE FORWARD TOGETHER

Your partner's cancer journey is now part of who you are as a couple. What does it mean for you now and in the future? Talk about it with your partner. Acknowledging the impact that cancer and its treatment has had on each of you can help you move forward.

While it's important to identify the challenges ahead, it's also important to celebrate the best parts of ending active treatment, of being able to withdraw from an intense medical environment into one that feels more like home, like you. You've made it through a tough time and you deserve to enjoy that. You might even consider marking the ending of treatment with a celebratory dinner or event, or a change of scenery like a vacation so you can come home with a fresh perspective.

14

Stopping anticancer treatment

When there's evidence the disease is progressing despite treatment, it's a reasonable choice to re-evaluate your next steps — similar to what you and your oncologist did when you first learned you had metastatic breast cancer and were deciding on treatment.

If the downsides of continuing cancer-directed treatment outweigh the potential benefits, it may be time to end active treatment. For example, for many people with cancer, there eventually comes a time when the chances that chemotherapy will make them sick — and maybe cause life-threatening side effects — are greater than the chances that it will shrink or control the cancer.

Deciding to end cancer-directed treatment is a personal decision you make, often with advice from your health care team, family and friends. Some people find it difficult to end treatment aimed at destroying or controlling cancer because it feels like they're giving up. But if cancer has become resistant to anticancer therapies, such treatments may do more harm than good. For many, quality of life takes center stage because they want to enjoy the time they have left.

You may feel as if your life has been out of control since you learned that you have metastatic cancer. Deciding to stop anticancer treatment that's no longer helping you may be a way for you to live life on your own terms again.

LEAVING A LEGACY

Even though we all eventually die, being forced to contemplate your mortality can be profoundly unsettling, especially at first. You may think not only of yourself, but also how the event of your death might impact your loved ones.

Some people with metastatic cancer have found healing and empowerment in creating a legacy by which others can remember them. This can be accomplished in different ways, such as:

- Writing down your life experiences or compiling a retrospective of your life and all you've accomplished.
- Creating a document, such as a family tree, detailing family health history; this can be especially important in families with genetic cancers.

- Making a video or audio recording in which you share life stories and special memories.
- Putting together a scrapbook of your favorite family moments.
- Creating a file filled with weekly notes to your children or other loved ones.
- Writing letters or making videos for important future events, such as graduations, weddings or the birth of a grandchild.
- Creating artwork that expresses your feelings on your life.
- Planting a garden with your favorite perennial flowers.
- Compiling a cookbook for your family and friends filled with recipes for your signature dishes and recipes you know to be favorites of your loved ones.
- Volunteering in the community or giving to a favorite charity.
- Getting involved in the metastatic breast cancer community, advocating for more metastatic cancer research funding or starting a nonprofit to help others with metastatic breast cancer.

There are multiple benefits to creating a legacy. For example, reviewing your family ties, accomplishments and life experiences can give you a sense of pride and a feeling that you've lived a full life. Life is limited for everyone, but not everyone has the chance to review it in a measured way. Doing so can bring some level of peace when you're facing an incurable illness.

If you're concerned about family and friends having to take care of you and support you, think about times when you were in a caregiving role. Reminiscing about raising children or caring for a loved one can relieve the feeling that you're a burden and soothe related distress. Talking about memories can sometimes improve feelings about others and your relationships with them. If those relationships have been strained recently, this could help bring peace and reconciliation.

HOSPICE CARE

If you've decided to stop cancer-directed treatments, management of your symptoms may continue through hospice care. Hospice is an insurance benefit covered by Medicare and many private insurance plans. As defined by Medicare, this benefit is for those who are expected to live six months or fewer. However, life expectancy is an estimate, and if people in hospice care live past six months, they can continue to receive services if their condition remains life-limiting.

The goal of hospice care is to manage symptoms and help you live as well as possible during the time you have remaining. It is also there — when the time comes — to help you die with peace and dignity. At all times, hospice provides support for your family and caregivers as well.

Most hospice care is provided at home, but hospice care may also be available in nursing homes and other residential settings. A few hospice programs have their own hospital or clinic facilities. As with general palliative care, hospice care is often provided by a team, large or small, that may include doctors, nurses, chaplains, social workers, volunteers and other professionals.

In a home setting, although nurses and other members of the hospice team make visits as needed, the program is designed so that the person who is dying receives much of their care from loved ones and can get advice and support from the hospice team 24 hours a day, seven days a week, whenever they need it.

Many people appreciate the benefits that home hospice care brings, including the freedom to be in familiar surroundings and away from an intense medical environment.

The services you receive may vary but can include:

- **Medications and supplies** Options for symptom management and physical equipment such as a hospital bed or walker may be provided.
- **Professional support** Hospice staff make regular visits to your home. They won't stay all day or night, but they are on call 24 hours a day, seven days a week. Staff can also deliver education for your caregivers.
- **Holistic well-being** Your team can help you address social, emotional or spiritual aspects of your care.
- **Breaks for caregivers** Hospice can provide respite care, which is short-term care to relieve the primary caregiver. Hospice volunteers can assist with basic tasks such as running errands and spending time with you or your family.
- **Bereavement support** These services are available to family members for 13 months after the death of a loved one.

Additional Resources

American Cancer Society
cancer.org

American Society of Clinical Oncologists
cancer.net

BreastCancer.org
breastcancer.org

Cancer Care
cancercare.org

findhelp.org
findhelp.org

Living Beyond Breast Cancer
lbbc.org

LiveStrong Foundation
livestrong.org

Mayo Clinic
mayoclinic.org

Mayo Clinic Comprehensive Cancer Center Blog
cancerblog.mayoclinic.org

Mayo Clinic Connect
connect.mayoclinic.org

Mayo Clinic Press Cancer Blog
mcpress.mayoclinic.org/cancer

National Cancer Institute
cancer.gov

Susan G. Komen Breast Cancer Foundation
komen.org

BLACK, INDIGENOUS AND PEOPLE OF COLOR

American Indian Cancer Foundation
americanindiancancer.org

Asian Women for Health
asianwomenforhealth.org

Chrysalis Initiative
thechrysalisinitiative.org

Coalition of Blacks Against Cancer
www.coalitionofblacksagainstcancer.org

Fight Through Flights
fightthroughflights.org

For the Breast of Us
breastofus.com

LatinaSHARE
latina.sharecancersupport.org

My Style Matters
https://mystylematters.org

TOUCH Black Breast Cancer Alliance
touchbbca.org

CAREER

Cancer and Careers
cancerandcareers.org

CHILDREN OF SURVIVORS

Brightspot Network
brightspotnetwork.org

Camp Kesem
kesem.org

CLINICAL TRIALS

ClinicalTrials.gov
clinicaltrials.gov

National Cancer Institute
cancer.gov/about-cancer/treatment/clinical-trials

FERTILITY

Chick Mission
thechickmission.org

FINANCES

Cancer Financial Assistance Coalition
https://www.cancerfac.org

Health Insurance Marketplace
healthcare.gov

Medicaid
medicaid.gov

Medicare (65+)
medicare.gov

NeedyMeds
needymeds.org

Social Security Disability Insurance (SSDI)
ssa.gov/benefits/disability/

State Health Insurance Assistance Program
shiphelp.org

Supplemental Security Income (SSI)
ssa.gov/ssi/

METASTATIC BREAST CANCER

Infinite Strength
infinitestrength.org

Project MBC Life
www.projectlifembc.com

Share Cancer Support
sharecancersupport.org

PATIENT ADVOCACY

Patient Advocate Foundation
https://www.Patientadvocate.org

Triage Cancer
triagecancer.org

YOUNG SURVIVORS

Stupid Cancer
stupidcancer.org

The Breasties
thebreasties.org

Tigerlily Foundation
tigerlilyfoundation.org

Young Survival Coalition
youngsurvival.org

These are only a few examples of organizations that offer support to breast cancer survivors. Note that eligibility requirements and availability of some of these resources can vary based on individual circumstances and geographic location. Consult with a social worker or patient navigator on your cancer care team or at your local hospital for help in navigating resources.

Index

A

acceptance, 105–106, 138

acupuncture. *See also*
   integrative therapies
   about, 121–122
   benefits of, 123–124
   how it works, 124
   for pain in treated breast
      area, 79
   risks and side effects, 125
   sessions, 124–125

adjuvant endocrine therapy,
   89

adoption, 157–158

advanced breast cancer.
   See metastatic breast
   cancer

alcohol use, avoiding/limiting,
   56–57, 82

Americans with Disabilities
   Act (ADA), 188–190

anger, 95–98, 158

anxiety, 19–20, 69–70, 72

appetite changes, 66–67

B

biofeedback, 79

body, rediscovering, 139

body image, boosting,
   138–140

body mass index (BMI),
   46–47

body scan meditation, 119

bone density testing, 58, 59

BRCA1 and BRCA2, 155, 170

breast MRI, 38

breast reconstruction, 35

breathing, 86, 117–118,
   120–121, 136

C

cancer care team, 14, 17, 23, 70,
   75, 85, 94

cancer screenings, 57–58

cancer survivors
  about, 15
  depression/anxiety and, 20
  fear and, 17
  finances and, 180–188
  online message boards for, 21
  post-traumatic growth and, 26
  support groups for, 20–21
  work return and, 174–180
  young, 213
cannabis, medical, 128–129
cardiovascular disease screening, 59–60
caregivers, 192–203. *See also* partners as caregivers
CBD, 128–130
cervical cancer screening, 57
chemotherapy, 80, 83, 93
children
  behavior in difficult circumstances, 105
  diagnosis communication with, 103–105
  explaining recovery to, 166
  fears of recurrence, helping manage, 169
  paying attention to, 167
  questions of, 166–167
  resources, 211
  spending extra time with, 168
  supporting, 165–168
clinical trials
  about, 111–112
  benefits of, 112
  finding, 114
  metastatic breast cancer and, 93–94
  participation in, 113–114
  phases, 112–113
  questions to ask, 115
  resources, 211
cognitive behavioral therapy for insomnia (CBT-I), 64–65
cognitive changes, 68–69
cognitive rehabilitation therapy, 69
colorectal cancer screening, 57
contraception, 147–150. *See also* reproductive health
co-workers, 178–179

D
dating after breast cancer, 142–145
depression, 19–20, 69–72, 98–99
diet, healthy, 43–46, 82
distant recurrence, 29, 31
donor sperm, 157
double barrier method, 148

E
eating guidelines, 44–45
echocardiogram, 60
egg donation, 156
emotions
  about, 14–16
  anger, 95–98, 158
  anxiety and, 19–20, 69–72
  coping with, 14–21, 158
  depression and, 19–20, 69–72, 98–99
  family life return and, 161
  fear and, 16–17
  infertility and, 158
  loneliness and, 20–21, 99
  stress and, 17–18, 54, 100, 160

endocrine therapy, 59, 83, 85, 87, 92
erectile dysfunction, 133, 137
exercise. *See* physical activity

F
family and friends
adjustment period, 173
cancer diagnosis communication with, 100–101
children and, 165–168
family life and, 160–165
family members cancer risk and, 170
reconnection with friends and, 168–173
Family and Medical Leave Act (FMLA), 190–191
family life, easing back into
about, 160
challenges, 160–162
changed roles/responsibilities and, 161
expectations and, 161–162
patience and, 162–163
priorities and, 163–164
team work and, 162–165
fatigue, 62–63
fear
coping with, 16–17
partner caregivers and, 198–199
recurrence, 16, 198
of rejection, 144–145
fertility. *See also* reproductive health
coping with emotions and, 158
IVF, 156
male survivors and, 153
options, 154–158

resources, 211
third-party options, 156–158
finances in survivorship
first steps, 181–182
medical costs, 183–188
metastatic breast cancer and, 182
navigators, 182
resources, 212
saving on meds and, 183
follow-up care
appointments, 28
doctor to see in, 22
oncologist visits and, 24
transitioning to, 22–24
friends, reconnecting with, 168–173. *See also* family and friends

G
Genetic Information Nondiscrimination Act (GINA), 191
gestational carrier, 156–157
government-sponsored insurance, 185
gratitude, 139, 164
grieving, 18–19, 95–98

H
health habits
about, 42–43
alcohol use and, 56–57
diet, 43–46
focusing on, 67
maximizing, 60
physical activity, 49–52
screenings and, 57–60
sleep, 52–54
smoking/vaping and, 54–56
weight, 46–49

hormonal contraceptives, 149
hormone therapy, 89
hospice care, 107–108,
    207–208
hypnosis, 127–189

I
immunotherapy, 93
insomnia, 64–66
integrative oncology, 109
integrative therapies
    about, 116
    acupuncture, 121–125
    hypnosis, 127–128
    massage, 125–127
    medical cannabis, 128–130
    mindfulness, 117–121
    uses of, 63, 65, 69, 82–83,
        84
intrauterine devices (IUDs),
    147, 148

L
legacy, 205–207
listening, 201
local recurrence, 29, 30, 33
loneliness, 20–21, 99, 169
loss, 18–19, 22. *See also*
    grieving
lubricants, 135, 136
lumpectomy, 29, 30, 34,
    36, 39
lung cancer screening, 58
lymphatic massage, 76
lymphedema
    about, 74–75
    early warning signs of, 75
    at-home treatment, 75–76
    infection risk, 78
    surgical treatment, 77
    therapy, 76–77

M
mammograms
    annual, 33–34
    breast reconstruction and,
        35
    contrast-enhanced imaging
        (CEM), 39–40
    men and, 36
    3-D, 39
manual lymph drainage, 126
massage therapy, 79, 125–127
mastectomy, local recurrence
    and, 30
medical costs, paying for,
    183–188. *See also* finances
    in survivorship
medical history, 48
Medicare and Medicaid, 185
meditation, 119–120
men with breast cancer
    changes in bodies, 87
    endocrine therapy and, 59,
        87
    fertility and, 153
    mammograms, 36
menopausal symptoms
    about, 84
    hormone therapy and, 89
    treatment for, 86–88
    types of, 85
metastatic breast cancer
    about, 90–91
    acceptance and, 105–106
    anger and, 95–98
    diagnosis communication,
        100–105
    emotions and coping,
        95–100
    finances and, 182
    forced positivity and,
        99–100

imaging tests and, 91
living with, 28
loneliness and, 99
physical activity and, 102
resources, 212–213
second opinions and, 96–97
treatment goals, 92, 94–95
treatment options, 92–94
metastatic recurrence, 29
mindfulness. *See also*
    integrative therapies
    about, 117–118
    caregivers and, 198
    exercises, 119–121
    therapies, 118–119
mindfulness-based stress
    reduction (MBSR), 118
muscle and joint pain, 83–84

N
natural family planning, 149
neuropathy, 80–83
noninvasive cancer, 32
nonprofits, 187–188
normal, "new," 24

O
oncologist, follow-up, 24, 25,
    28
osteoporosis screening, 58
ovarian damage, 152
ovarian suppression drugs,
    150

P
pain/discomfort
    muscle and joint pain,
        83–84
    phantom, 81
    in treated breast area,
        79–80

vaginal, sex and, 134–137
palliative care
    about, 107
    benefits of, 110
    examples of, 108
    hospice care vs., 107–108
    insurance and, 108
    locations for, 110
    quality of life and,
        107–108
partner
    body image and, 139
    cancer diagnosis and,
        101–103
    reconnecting with,
        140–142
partners as caregivers
    about, 192–193
    allowing for struggle and,
        200
    connection and, 200
    fear and, 198–199
    listening and, 201
    mindfulness and, 198
    personal story, 202
    physical needs, 194
    processing time and,
        193–194
    psychological needs, 196
    roles/responsibilities and,
        201
    self-care, 194–200
    sex and, 201
    spirituality and, 199–200
    support for each other and,
        200–203
patient advocacy resources,
    213
phantom breast pain, 81
phases of clinical trials,
    112–113

physical activity. *See also* health habits
  benefits of, 49–50
  body image and, 138
  fatigue and, 62–63
  metastatic breast cancer and, 102
  neuropathy and, 81
  recommendations, 50–51
  sleep and, 53
  starting, 51–52
  weight gain/loss and, 67
physical therapy, 79, 84
positivity, forced, 99–100
post-traumatic growth, 26
pregnancy (after cancer). *See also* reproductive health
  about, 150–151
  baby health and, 154
  common questions about, 151
  likelihood of, 151–152
  safety, 152–154
primary cancer, 28, 29
private insurance, 184–185
psychological needs, 196–197
psychotherapy, 63, 70

Q
qigong, 121
quit-smoking products, 56

R
recurrence, cancer
  categories of, 29
  children fears of, 169
  distant, 29, 31
  eating soy and, 47
  local, 29, 30, 33
  new cancer vs., 29
  regional, 29, 30

  treating, 41
  uncertainty and, 40–41
  understanding, 28–36
regional recurrence, 29, 30
relaxation exercises, 54
renewal, 14
reproductive health
  about, 146–147
  contraception and, 147–150
  fertility and, 154–158
  pregnancy and, 150–154
resources
  Black, indigenous and people of color, 210–211
  career, 211
  children of survivors, 211
  clinical trials, 211
  fertility, 211
  finances, 212
  general, 209–210
  metastatic breast cancer, 212–213
  patient advocacy, 213
risk reducing medicine, surveillance visits and, 31–32
romance, 141

S
savings accounts, 187
scarring, 72–74
screenings
  annual mammograms, 33–34
  breast MRI, 38
  cancer, 57–58
  contrast-enhanced mammography (CEM), 39–40
  guidelines for, 27–28
  health habits and, 57–60

molecular breast imaging (MBI), 38
recommended, 32–34
regular checkup, 32–33
routine health, 58
supplemental, 37–40
3-D mammogram, 39
treatment-related, 58–60
second opinions, 96–97
self-compassion, 144
sex therapists, 142
sexual experimentation, 141
sexual health
about, 131–132
body image and, 138–140
changes from treatments, 132–134
dating and, 142–145
erectile dysfunction and, 133, 137
orgasm/foreplay and, 133–134
reconnecting with partner and, 140–142
sexual desire and, 133
vaginal wall changes and, 132
wellness, restoring, 134–137
sexual pleasure, 141–142
shoulder and arm movement, restricted, 77–78
side effects
about, 61–62
anxiety and depression, 69–72
breast area discomfort/pain, 79–80
cognitive changes, 68–69
endocrine therapy, 85
fatigue, 62–63
general, 62–72
insomnia, 64–66
of local or regional treatment, 72
lymphedema, 74–77
menopausal symptoms and sexual changes, 84–88
muscle and joint pain, 83–84
neuropathy, 80–83
restricted shoulder and arm movement, 77–78
scarring, 72–73
of systemic treatments, 80–88
weight/appetite changes, 66–67
sitting meditation, 120
sleep, 52–54, 64–66
sleep aids, 65–66
SMART goals, 48–49
smoking/vaping, 54–56, 82
social security disability insurance (SSDI), 186–187
soy, eating, 47
spirituality, 122–123, 199–200
stage IV cancer. See metastatic breast cancer
sterilization, 149
stress, 17–18, 54, 100, 160
supplemental insurance, 187
supplemental screening, 37–40
supplements, dietary, 43–46
supplements, for insomnia, 66
support, from cancer care team, 14
support groups, 20–21
supportive care treatments, 94

surveillance, cancer
about, 27–28
frequency of visits, 31–32
recommended screening,
32–36
tests that aren't recom-
mended, 34–36
what to watch for,
30–31
survivorship care plan, 23
systemic treatment side
effects, 80–88

T
tai chi, 120–121
targeted therapy, 93
tax benefits, 188
tests, not recommended,
34–36
transition from treatment,
13–14, 22–24
treatment, cancer
ending, 204–208
metastatic breast cancer,
91–95
questions after, 25
recovery from, 15–16
sexual health changes and,
132–134
side effects, 61–89
transitioning from, 13–14
treatment, stopping
about, 204–205
hospice care and, 207–208

leaving a legacy and,
205–207
treatment-related screenings,
58–60

V
vaginal pain, 134–137

W
waist circumference, 47–48
walking meditation, 120
weight, healthy, 46–49, 67. *See
also* health habits
weight changes, 66–67
work return
about, 174–175
accommodations, 177–178
ADA and, 188–190
coworkers and, 178–179
FMLA and, 190–191
knowing rights and,
188–191
reluctance, 175–177
schedule adjustments,
177–178
self-consciousness and,
176–177
working from home and,
178

Y
yoga, 120
young cancer survivor
resources, 213

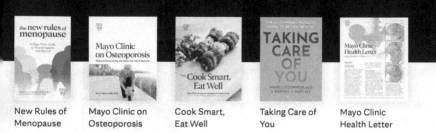